C

THE NEW BIBLE

CURE

FOR DIABETES

DON COLBERT, MD

SILOAM

Most CHARISMA HOUSE BOOK GROUP products are available at special quantity discounts for bulk purchase for sales promotions, premiums, fund-raising, and educational needs. For details, write Charisma House Book Group, 600 Rinehart Road, Lake Mary, Florida 32746, or telephone (407) 333-0600.

THE NEW BIBLE CURE FOR DIABETES by Don Colbert, MD
Published by Siloam
Charisma Media/Charisma House Book Group
600 Rinehart Road, Lake Mary, Florida 32746
www.charismahouse.com

Library of Congress Cataloging in Publication:
Colbert, Don.
   The new Bible cure for diabetes / by Don Colbert. -- [Rev. and expanded].
     p. cm.
   "Portions ... were previously published as The Bible cure for diabetes"--T.p. verso.
   Includes bibliographical references and index.
   ISBN 978-1-59979-759-5
  1. Diabetes--Popular works. 2. Diabetes--Alternative treatment. 3. Diabetes--Religious aspects--Christianity. I. Colbert, Don. Bible cure for diabetes. II. Title.
   RC660.4.C65 2009
   616.4'62--dc22
                         2009032276

E-book ISBN: 978-1-61638-017-5
Available at Amazon

11 12 13 14 — 11 10 9 8
Printed in the United States of America

CONTENTS

INTRODUCTION
  A NEW BIBLE CURE WITH
  NEW HOPE FOR DIABETES..............................1
  Diabetes Is a "Choice" Disease 3

1 KNOW YOUR ENEMY 7
  Different Types of Diabetes.................................. 8
    Type 1 diabetes 8
    Type 2 diabetes 11
    Gestational diabetes............................... 15
  Metabolic Syndrome.. 16
  Stress and Diabetes... 17
  Symptoms You Must Not Ignore 18
  Treatable and Beatable 19
  The Long-Term Complications of Diabetes
  (Termites)... 20
  The Good News.. 26

2 BATTLE DIABETES WITH GOOD
  NUTRITION 29
  Your Waistline Is Your Lifeline............................. 29
  What Is the Glycemic Index?.............................. 31
  The Glycemic Load 33
  The Bible and Fats.. 37

Fantastic Fiber 39

A Word of Caution.................................... 41

What About Bread?.................................. 42

A Final Word 45

3 BATTLE DIABETES WITH ACTIVITY.............49

Aerobic Activity 51

Resistance Exercises................................ 53

Sticking With It... 54

Now, Take the Offensive!........................ 55

4 BATTLE DIABETES WITH WEIGHT LOSS.......59

A Powerful Key to Prevention................. 59

Your Ideal Weight—Catch the Vision! 60

Dr. Colbert's Rapid Waist Reduction Diet............ 62

Allowable foods 62

Foods to limit or avoid 65

Treats and cheats (for weekends only;
best to eat before 3:00 p.m.; commit to this
program for thirty days before cheating)............ 66

Simple Rules... 66

Faith Moves Mountains 68

5 BATTLE DIABETES WITH NUTRIENTS AND SUPPLEMENTS...............73

A good multivitamin 73

Vitamin D.. 75

Chromium... 75

Alpha lipoic acid 79

Cinnamon 80

Soluble fiber... 81

Irvingia... 83

Omega-3 fatty acids... 84

Supplements to Decrease Glycation 85

Carnosine 85

Pyridoxamine.. 85

Benfotiamine 86

Supplements to Replenish Hormones 87

Testosterone... 88

Estrogen 90

Progesterone.. 90

A Final Note 91

6 BATTLE DIABETES WITH SPIRITUAL AND EMOTIONAL STRENGTH 95

Another Dimension... 95

Less Stress... 96

Take These Bible Cure Steps 97

Enjoy the present moment. 97

Reframe your thinking.. 98

Build margin into your life. 98

Remove obvious stressors, and
surround yourself with positive people............... 99

Learn the power of "no." 99

Pray... 100

Meditate on God's Word.................................. 100

A PERSONAL NOTE From Don Colbert 103

APPENDIX
NUTRITIONAL SUPPLEMENTS
FOR DIABETES 105

NOTES.. 107

A NEW BIBLE CURE WITH NEW HOPE FOR DIABETES

G OD'S DESIRE IS for you to feel better and to live longer, and He will help you reach that goal! By picking up this revised and expanded Bible Cure book, you have taken an exciting first step toward renewed energy, health, and vigor.

You may be confronting the greatest physical challenge of your life. But with faith in God and good nutrition, combined with cutting-edge alternative natural remedies, I believe it will be your greatest victory! God revealed His divine will for each of us through the apostle John, who wrote, "Beloved, I pray that you may prosper in all things and be in health, just as your soul prospers" (3 John 2, NKJV).

Nearly two thousand years later, almost 24 million Americans suffer from a disease called diabetes—and a fourth of them don't even know they have it! Diabetes kills more people than AIDS and breast cancer combined and reportedly ranks as the sixth leading cause of death by disease among adults in America.[1] The sad reality is that it may rank much higher because research shows that diabetes is underreported as a cause of death. Studies have found that diabetes was only listed as an underlying cause of death on 10 to 15 percent of death certificates when the decedent suffered from the disease.[2]

The World Health Organization (WHO) estimates that by 2030, the number of individuals with diabetes worldwide will double. That means we could see the number of people suffering from diabetes worldwide reach as high as 360 million within the next twenty years.[3]

Within the United States, type 2 diabetes is increasing at an alarming rate. Approximately one out of ten Americans age twenty and older has diabetes.[4] And the number of children being diagnosed with type 2 diabetes is growing at an alarming rate as well. Researchers at the Centers for Disease Control and Prevention (CDC) recently made the stunning prediction that without changes in diet and exercise, one in three children born in the United States in 2000 are likely to develop type 2 diabetes at some point in their lives. The prediction was especially serious for Latino children, whose odds of developing diabetes as they grow older were about fifty-fifty.[5]

Why are we seeing such an increase in diabetes? It is simply the result of the obesity epidemic: two-thirds of American adults are overweight or obese, and one-fifth of children in the United States are overweight.[6]

Surely we are missing God's best for us. But how? Many physicians are looking for the next new-and-improved medicine in order to treat diabetes. Instead, we need to get to the *root* of the problem, which is our diet, lifestyle, and waistline.

Fast food, junk food, convenience foods, sodas, sweetened coffee drinks, juices, smoothies, large portion sizes, and skipping meals are all pieces of the problem. The standard American diet is also full of empty carbohydrates, sugars, fats, excessive proteins, excessive calories, and large portion sizes, and it is quite low in nutrient content. This diet literally causes us to lose nutrients such as chromium, which is very important in glucose regulation.

Lack of activity is another piece of the problem. Most children are no longer playing sports and participating in other activities but are instead hooked on video games, computers, text messaging, TV shows, and movies as they gain more and more weight in the process.

Also, the excessive stress that most adults and many children are under is increasing cortisol levels, and, as a result, many are developing toxic belly fat, which increases the risk of diabetes. Long-term stress also depletes stress hormones as well as neurotransmitters, which usually unleash a ravenous appetite as well as addictions to sugar and carbohydrates.

Diabetes Is a "Choice" Disease

Galatians 6:7–8 says, "Do not be deceived, God is not mocked; for whatever a man sows, that he will also reap. For he who sows to his flesh will of the flesh reap corruption, but he who sows to the Spirit will of the Spirit reap everlasting life" (NKJV). Most Americans are unknowingly sowing seeds for a harvest of obesity, diabetes, and a host of other diseases by their choices of food and lifestyle habits.

I often say that prediabetes and type 2 diabetes are "choice" diseases. In other words, you *catch* a cold or you *catch* the flu, but you *develop* obesity, prediabetes, and type 2 diabetes as a result of wrong choices.

Hosea 4:6 says, "My people are destroyed for lack of knowledge" (NKJV). My books *The Seven Pillars of Health* and *Eat This and Live!* and my new weight-loss book, *Dr. Colbert's "I Can*

Do This" Diet, provide a good foundation for changing dietary patterns, improving lifestyle habits, and losing weight—especially the toxic belly fat that is so closely related to diabetes.

In this book, you will learn about natural ways to avoid and reverse diabetes, but you will also learn the different types of diabetes, how it develops, and the terrible complications of diabetes as it damages and may eventually destroy the kidneys, eventually leading to dialysis. It also damages the blood vessels and may lead to blindness, impotence, heart attack, stroke, and poor circulation in the extremities. It also damages nerves, leading to burning pains in the feet (like someone is constantly burning you with cigarettes), numbness in the feet, foot and leg ulcers, infections, and possibly eventual amputation.

Now you are getting the picture as you are beginning to realize that when you habitually drink soda or eat that piece of cake, pie, candy bar, or large helping of white rice, potatoes, and white bread that you are unknowingly signing up for prediabetes and diabetes.

I have seen patients over the years stressed out over signing a contract without reading the small print. Recently, a patient came in who was very upset because after moving out of his apartment, he found out that he owed the apartment complex an extra one thousand dollars. He said that he never had to do that before after moving out of other apartments. They had informed him to simply read his contract. He did, and it said in very fine print that when the occupant of the apartment moved out, a payment of one thousand dollars would be required.

Most Americans are unknowingly signing on the dotted line for a harvest of diabetes accompanied by all of the complications associated with the disease. Wake up while there is still time to reverse the curse of diabetes and prediabetes!

You may be wondering if there is any hope, and I am here to tell you there is! You see, your body is fearfully and wonderfully made, and regardless of which type of diabetes you or a loved one may have, God can totally heal either one without effort or difficulty. I've known some people who have been completely healed of diabetes by the miracle-working power of God. I have also witnessed many others whose lives have been dramatically improved through healthy lifestyle choices and natural treatments. Realize that God generally won't do what you can do. Only you can choose to eat healthy foods, exercise, lose weight, and take supplements.

Since the original publication of *The Bible Cure for Diabetes* in 1999, many new things about diabetes have come to light, and many of the terms used to identify this illness have changed. *The New Bible Cure for Diabetes* has been revised and updated to reflect the latest medical research on diabetes. If you compare it side by side with the previous edition, you'll see that it's also larger, allowing me to expand greatly upon the information provided in the previous edition and provide you with a deeper understanding of what you face and how to overcome it.

Unchanged from the previous edition are the timeless, life-changing, and healing scriptures throughout this book that will strengthen and encourage your spirit and soul. The proven principles, truths, and guidelines in these passages anchor the practical and medical insights also contained in this book. They will effectively focus your prayers, thoughts, and actions so you can step into God's plan of divine health for you—a plan that includes victory over diabetes.

Another change since the original *The Bible Cure for Diabetes* was published is that I've released a foundational book, *The Seven Pillars of Health.* I encourage you to read it because the principles of health it contains are the foundation to healthy living that will affect all areas of your life. It sets the stage for everything you will ever read in any other book I've published—including this one.

There is much we can do to prevent or defeat diabetes. Now it is time to run to the battle with fresh confidence, renewed determination, and the wonderful knowledge that God is real, He is alive, and His power is greater than any sickness or disease.

It is my prayer that these practical suggestions for health, nutrition, and fitness will bring wholeness to your life. May they deepen your fellowship with God and strengthen your ability to worship and serve Him.

—DON COLBERT, MD

A BIBLE CURE *Prayer for You*

Dear heavenly Father, You have declared in Your Word that I am healed by the stripes Your Son, Jesus Christ, bore on His back. For Your Word says, "He was pierced for our rebellion, crushed for our sins. He was beaten so we could be whole. He was whipped so we could be healed" (Isa. 53:5).

Father, Your Son, Jesus, has given us the authority to use His name when we pray. This is the same name by which You spoke into being the heavens and the earth long ago. In that precious name I declare that Your Word is true: I am healed by the whipping Jesus bore on His back. Whether I must wait for a minute, a week, a year, or a lifetime for my physical healing to be complete, by faith I will praise You for it as if it were already complete. I thank You for a healthy pancreas that produces and properly regulates the insulin levels in my body. Amen.

1

KNOW YOUR ENEMY

THOUSANDS OF YEARS ago, the Romans and Greeks had some understanding of diabetes even though they had no blood test for diabetes back then. It might surprise you to learn that the Romans and Greeks were able to detect diabetes by simply tasting a person's urine. It's true! They discovered that some people's urine had a sweet taste, or *mellitus*, which is the Latin word for "sweet." Also, the Greeks realized that when patients with sweet urine drank any fluids, the fluids were generally excreted in the urine almost as rapidly as they went in the mouth, similar to a siphon. The Greek word for "siphon" is *diabetes*. So now you know how we got the name diabetes mellitus: it all started by tasting the urine. I for one am glad that doctors abandoned this practice centuries ago and that now we simply check a patient's blood sugar!

I have good news for you too: Not only is this disease thousands of years old, but so is God's power to heal. God healed the sick thousands of years ago in the days of the Bible, and He still heals today! He has also given us a wealth of proven Bible principles and invaluable medical knowledge about the human body. You can control the symptoms and potentially damaging effects of diabetes while you seek Him for total healing. You are destined to be more than a victim. You are destined to be a victor in this battle!

Your first order of battle is to *know your enemy*. Measure its strengths, and plan for its defeat. The enemy called diabetes comes in various forms.

DIFFERENT TYPES OF DIABETES

Diabetes is actually a group of diseases including type 1 diabetes, type 2 diabetes, and gestational diabetes. Each type of diabetes is characterized by high levels of blood sugar that is the result of either defects in insulin production, defects in the action of insulin, or both.

As I said in the introduction of this book, a person does not just wake up one day with type 2 diabetes. Developing type 2 diabetes is a slow, insidious process that usually takes years to a decade to develop. It always starts with prediabetes.

Prediabetes (formerly called *borderline* or *subclinical diabetes*) is defined as a blood sugar level of 100 to 125 mg/dL (milligrams per deciliter) after an eight-hour fast. Prediabetes is also defined as a blood sugar level of 140 to 199 mg/dL two hours after eating. A normal fasting blood sugar level is less than 100 mg/dL, and a normal blood sugar level two hours after eating is less than 140 mg/dL.[1]

Diabetes is defined as a fasting blood sugar level greater than or equal to 126 mg/dL or a casual blood sugar level (usually after eating) greater than or equal to 200 mg/dL. High blood sugar levels are accompanied by symptoms of diabetes, including frequent urination, excessive thirst, and changes in vision.[2]

Type 1 diabetes

In the past, type 1 diabetes has been called insulin-dependent diabetes, juvenile-onset diabetes, or childhood-onset diabetes.

This form of diabetes usually occurs in children or young adults, although it can strike at any age. In adults, it is quite rare with only about 5 to 10 percent of all cases of diabetes being type 1 diabetes.[3]

We currently do not have all the pieces of the puzzle for type 1 diabetes, but risk factors may be genetic or environmental. Some researchers believe that the environmental trigger is probably a virus. Others believe the trigger may be ingesting cow's milk protein, especially during infancy.

What we *do* know is that type 1 diabetes is caused by the body's own immune system attacking itself and eventually destroying the beta cells in the pancreas. The beta cells are the only cells in the body that make insulin, which is the hormone that regulates blood sugar. Patients with type 1 diabetes require insulin either by injection or by an insulin pump in order to survive.

Over the years, I have found that my patients who have maintained the best blood sugar control have been the patients using the insulin pump. The newer insulin pumps actually have remote controls, making it much easier to control the blood sugar. I have also discovered that dietary and lifestyle changes and nutritional supplements will usually lower insulin requirements in type 1 diabetics. It is very important to monitor your blood sugar daily and to adjust your insulin accordingly once beginning this program. Also, have your doctor monitor you on a regular basis.

The hemoglobin A1C test is the best way to monitor your blood sugar over the long run. Hemoglobin is a protein that carries oxygen in the blood and is present inside the red blood cells that live only for about ninety to one hundred twenty days.

The hemoglobin A1C measures how much glucose has entered the red blood cells and become stuck to the hemoglobin, similar to a fly stuck to flypaper.[4]

If a person usually has a high blood sugar level throughout the day, more sugar will be stuck to the hemoglobin, but if the blood sugar is typically only slightly elevated during the day, less sugar will be stuck to the hemoglobin, and the hemoglobin A1C will be lower.

Most diabetes specialists recommend that diabetic patients get their hemoglobin A1C to 6.5 percent or lower in order to prevent most of the complications of diabetes. They also recommend that the diabetic patients check this blood test approximately every three to four months. I personally try to get my diabetic patients hemoglobin A1C to around 6 percent because at this level, I find that they rarely ever develop severe complications of diabetes.

Individuals battling with type 1 diabetes will also greatly benefit from the nutritional information and biblical truths shared in this book. Continue to follow all of the advice of your physician, and consult him or her before making any lifestyle and nutritional changes. In addition, determine to believe God—who created your pancreas in the first place—for a miraculous touch of healing power. The Word of God says, "For nothing is impossible with God" (Luke 1:37).

> Don't you realize that all of you together are the
> temple of God and that the Spirit of God lives in you?
> God will destroy anyone who destroys this temple.
> For God's temple is holy, and you are that temple.
>   —1 CORINTHIANS 3:16–17

Remember that faith is not a feeling or an emotion; faith is a choice. Specifically ask the Lord to heal your pancreas and restore its ability to manufacture insulin.

Type 2 diabetes

Type 2 diabetes was previously called non-insulin-dependent diabetes or adult-onset diabetes because historically people contracted the disease in their adult years. However, our nation's taste for a high-sugar, high-fat diet seems to have removed the age barrier. The medical community now reports that this form of diabetes accounts for a growing number of juvenile cases. In adults, 90 to 95 percent of all diabetes cases are type 2 diabetes. In other words, nine to nine and a half cases out of every ten cases of diabetes are type 2.[5] According to the National Institutes of Health, 1.6 million new cases of diabetes in people age twenty and older were diagnosed in 2007.[6]

Type 2 diabetes is more of a genetic disease than type 1 diabetes. However, before you blame your genes for this disease, understand this: your genetic makeup may have "loaded the gun," but environmental factors, such as belly fat, poor diet, and lifestyle factors, will "pull the trigger."

In other words, many people might have the genetic predisposition for type 2 diabetes; however, if they lose belly fat, control their diets, and exercise regularly, they will probably never develop diabetes. In fact, a large diabetes prevention study found that lifestyle changes reduced developing diabetes by more than 70 percent in high-risk people who were over sixty years old.[7]

The majority of people with type 2 diabetes still produces insulin; however, the cells in their bodies do not use the insulin properly. This condition is known as insulin resistance. Over time, insulin resistance leads to prediabetes and type 2 diabetes.

For years, I have explained to patients that insulin is like a key that unlocks the door to your cells, and having type 2 diabetes is similar to having rusty locks on those cells. Every cell in your body needs sugar, and the hormone insulin removes sugar from the bloodstream and binds to insulin receptors on the surface of the cells, very similar to a key unlocking a lock and opening the door. The insulin opens the door to the cells (figuratively speaking) and allows sugar to enter in.

However, in type 2 diabetics, the cells resist the normal function of insulin. In other words, the key goes in to unlock the lock, but, similar to a rusty lock, the insulin does not work as well. If you have ever tried to open an old, rusty lock, you will understand this analogy.

Insulin levels then begin to rise as more and more insulin is needed to allow sugar to enter into the cells. This is very similar to jiggling the key over and over until the key unlocks the rusty lock. That means that an excessive amount of insulin is needed to keep the blood sugar level in the normal range. Eventually, as cells become more and more insulin resistant, higher insulin levels are unable to lower the blood sugar. The blood sugar begins to rise higher and higher as the person develops prediabetes and eventually type 2 diabetes. Usually patients with prediabetes have no symptoms.

As this stage of insulin resistance worsens, a person will eventually develop prediabetes, which is defined as having fasting blood sugars greater than 100 mg/dL and less than 126 mg/dL. People with prediabetes typically have impaired glucose tolerance (IGT), impaired fasting glucose (IFG), or both. Often they do not know they have prediabetes because there are no symptoms initially. It typically takes years, sometimes even more than a decade, to progress from prediabetes into full-blown type 2 diabetes.

By the time people develop type 2 diabetes, they typically experience symptoms such as increased thirst, increased urination, nighttime urination, blurry vision, or fatigue. Type 2 diabetes is typically associated with obesity (especially truncal obesity), older age, a family history of diabetes, physical inactivity, or a history of gestational diabetes. Race also plays a role in risk for the disease: American Indians, Hispanic Americans, African Americans, and some Asian Americans and Pacific Islanders have a higher risk of developing type 2 diabetes and its complications.

Insulin resistance is one of the greatest health enemies of people suffering from type 2 diabetes. This is usually a very manageable problem, but it is complicated by the fact that truncal obesity is one of the most important factors leading to insulin resistance. That means that obese people with type 2 diabetes must fight a battle on two fronts: they must drop their weight down to safer levels while they also carefully monitor and control their blood sugar levels. This also means that type 2 diabetics require:

- A diet that is low in refined, processed starches such as white rice, white bread, potatoes, and pasta
- A diet that has very little sugar

A **BIBLE CURE** Health Tip
High-Fructose Corn Syrup: Sugar in Disguise

If you have diabetes, you undoubtedly have been told how important it is to limit the amount of sugar in your diet. You know you need to choose your foods carefully, but food manufacturers can be sneaky. Don't forget to watch out for one of sugar's many aliases: high-fructose corn syrup (HFCS).

HFCS is a blend of glucose and fructose. Glucose, obviously, is the form of sugar in your blood that you monitor as a diabetic. Fructose is the primary carbohydrate in most fruits. Well, if it's from fruit, it's healthy, right? Not exactly. While it is fine to consume small amounts of fructose because your body metabolizes it differently and it does not trigger your body's appetite control center, consuming large amounts sets you up for unhealthy weight gain.

Since HFCS is in many commercial food and drink products, I highly recommend that you stick to the outer aisles at the grocery store and purchase fresh produce, whole grains, and lean meats. Avoid the center aisles, and you will be well on your way to avoiding the risk of consuming a "stealth" sugar that's hidden in a packaged, processed food product. Many researchers believe that America's excessive intake of HFCS is responsible for our diabetes epidemic.

HFCS represents 40 percent of calorie sweeteners added to foods and beverages and is the only sweeteners in soft drinks in the United States. Now America consumes about sixty pounds a year of HFCS. The liver metabolizes fructose into fat more readily than it does glucose. Consuming HFCS can lead to a nonalcoholic fatty liver, which usually precedes insulin resistance and type 2 diabetes. If HFCS is one of the first ingredients on the food label, don't eat or drink it. Here is a list of foods that are high in HFCS:

- Soft drinks
- Popsicles
- Pancake syrup
- Frozen yogurt
- Breakfast cereals
- Canned fruits
- Fruit-flavored yogurt
- Ketchup and barbecue sauce
- Pasta sauces in jars and cans
- Fruit drinks that are not 100 percent fruit

Gestational diabetes

Gestational diabetes is a form of diabetes acquired during pregnancy and only occurs in about 2 percent of pregnancies. Gestational diabetes is due to the growing fetus and placenta secreting hormones that decrease the body's sensitivity to insulin and can cause diabetes.

If a woman does contract gestational diabetes, it usually goes away after giving birth. Only 5 to 10 percent of women with gestational diabetes are found to have type 2 diabetes after giving birth. However, it does increase a woman's risk of developing type 2 diabetes later in life. Studies show that 40 to 60 percent of women who developed gestational diabetes will develop type 2 diabetes within five to ten years after pregnancy. Gestational diabetes occurs more frequently among African Americans, American Indians, and Hispanic Americans.

METABOLIC SYNDROME

Many individuals who have prediabetes and type 2 diabetes also have metabolic syndrome (formerly called syndrome X). Metabolic syndrome is simply a group of risk factors, and the more of these risk factors you have, the higher your risk of heart disease, stroke, and diabetes.

You have metabolic syndrome if you have at least three of the following criteria:

- A waist measurement greater than 40 inches for men or 35 inches for women
- High blood pressure (130/85 or greater)
- Fasting blood sugar of 100 mg/dL or greater
- Triglyceride level of 150 mg/dL or greater
- Low HDL (good) cholesterol (below 40 mg/dL for men or 50 mg/dL for women)

Almost 25 percent of American adults have metabolic syndrome. Chances of developing metabolic syndrome are closely linked to overweight, obesity, and an inactive lifestyle.[8]

STRESS AND DIABETES

Excessive stress can increase glucose levels in patients with diabetes, predisposing them to long-term complications, including kidney disease, eye disease, neuropathy, and vascular disease.

In one study, diabetic patients were randomly involved in education sessions with and without stress management training. The stress management training included progressive muscle relaxation, breathing techniques, and mental imagery. All participants were at least thirty years of age and managing their diabetes with diet, exercise, and/or non-insulin medications.[9]

At the end of one year, 32 percent of the patients in the stress management group had hemoglobin A1C levels that were lowered by 1 percent or more. Hemoglobin A1C is a standard blood test used to determine average blood sugar levels over a period of a few months. Lowering hemoglobin A1C by 1 percent is considered very significant, and stress management did this in one-third of the patients. However, only 12 percent of the control subjects had hemoglobin A1C levels that were lowered by this much.[10]

Stress reduction is very important in helping to control diabetes since high cortisol levels, which is the main stress hormone, is also associated with increased belly fat, elevations of blood sugar, and increased insulin levels. I teach numerous stress-reduction techniques in my book *Stress Less*. I strongly recommend you read this book.

SYMPTOMS YOU MUST NOT IGNORE

As with most diseases, early detection of diabetes is very important. Silent enemies sometimes inflict the most damage. Fortunately, type 2 diabetes has some telltale symptoms that may tip you off to a problem that needs attention:

- Urinary frequency and nighttime urination
- Increased hunger and thirst
- Feelings of edginess, fatigue, or nausea
- Blurred vision
- Tingling, numbness, or loss of feeling in the hands or feet
- Dry, itchy skin
- Sores that don't heal
- Repeated or hard-to-heal infections of the skin, gums, vagina, or bladder
- Loss of hair on the feet and lower legs

Some of these symptoms may occur from time to time simply because you drink too much liquid one night, eat some spicy food, or stay up too late. However, if you experience one or more of these symptoms on a regular basis, make an appointment with your physician, and get screened for diabetes and prediabetes. Then you can apply the truths in this book and in God's Word to the situation. Above all, don't give in to fear or apathy.

TREATABLE AND BEATABLE

As with most diseases, serious health complications occur when someone with diabetes fails to do anything about this treatable and beatable disease. The more serious complications of diabetes include diabetic retinopathy (the leading cause of blindness in the United States), diabetic neuropathy (a degeneration of peripheral nerves that leads to tingling, numbness, pain, and weakness usually in extremities such as the legs and feet), kidney disease, and arteriosclerosis (a narrowing of the arteries due to fatty deposits on the artery walls).

> Then God said, "Look! I have given you every seed-bearing plant throughout the earth and all the fruit trees for your food. And I have given every green plant as food for all the wild animals, the birds in the sky, and the small animals that scurry along the ground—everything that has life." And that is what happened.
>
> —GENESIS 1:29–30

Diabetics—particularly those who fail to control their insulin and blood sugar levels through proper diet, exercise, and lifestyle choices—are much more prone to heart disease, heart attacks, kidney disease (one of the main causes of death in diabetics), diabetic foot ulcers (usually due to a poor blood supply), and peripheral nerve disease of the feet.

THE LONG-TERM COMPLICATIONS OF DIABETES (TERMITES)

Most people with diabetes think that they will never develop long-term complications of the disease. They rationalize that they will surely have early signs and symptoms before they develop these terrible complications of diabetes, or they assume they will be able to take medications that will reverse these diseases.

I often tell people that diabetes is very similar to a house with termites, and when termites have been eating away at a home for years, one day when you try to hang a picture on a wall, a gaping hole may suddenly appear, or your door may get stuck, and as you push on the door, the door frame may cave in. Now, this does not happen immediately with termites but with months or years of termite infestation.

Poorly controlled diabetes is a silent killer that works very similarly to termites. After years or decades, terrible health conditions suddenly begin to occur as a result of long-term diabetes. Medications can slow the process or control symptoms but usually do not get to the root of the problem.

The National Institutes of Health (NIH) say that diabetes contributes to the following diseases and health complications:

- *Vascular disease.* Individuals with poorly controlled long-term diabetes are also at a much greater risk of developing vascular disease (disease of the blood vessels). Long-term elevated blood sugar eventually accelerates plaque formation in all arteries of the body. As plaque accumulates in the coronary arteries from diabetes, people are more prone to develop heart disease or suffer a heart attack.

- Many diabetics suffer heart attacks, and due to the neuropathy, they may not experience the typical severe chest pain associated with heart attacks. Some actually experience silent heart attacks, where they feel no pain at all.

- Another type of vascular disease caused by diabetes is peripheral vascular disease, or clogging of the arteries, especially in the feet and legs. Many long-term diabetics can no longer feel their pulse in their feet, or they experience *claudication* (pain in the calves with walking that subsides with rest), both of which are symptoms of peripheral vascular disease.

- Long-term diabetics who smoke and have hypertension and high cholesterol are at a much greater risk of developing peripheral vascular disease. Fish oil, aspirin, and medications, along with aggressive risk factor modification such as blood sugar control, are usually needed to help people with peripheral vascular disease.[11]

- *Stroke.* A stroke is sometimes called a heart attack of the brain. Diabetics are very prone to plaque buildup in the arteries that supply blood to the brain, putting them at an increased risk of stroke. A diabetic may have a TIA (transient ischemic attack) in which he develops slurring of the speech, numbness, or weakness on one side of the body that usually goes away after a few hours. Having a TIA is a very ominous sign of an impending stroke, and you should go to the emergency room or see your physician immediately if you experience this.[12]

- *High blood pressure.* An estimated 73 percent of adults with diabetes also have high blood pressure or are taking medications for hypertension.[13] The cause should be obvious, considering the effects of diabetes on the cardiovascular and circulatory system mentioned earlier.

- *Eye disease.* Long-term diabetes also affects the eyes and may lead to diabetic retinopathy, loss of vision, and eventual blindness. Diabetic retinopathy is a common condition seen in diabetics who have had the disease for more than ten years. Between 40 and 45 percent of people with diabetes have some stage of diabetic retinopathy.[14] Diabetic retinopathy causes up to twenty-four thousand new cases of blindness every year.[15]

- Without good blood sugar control, numerous changes occur in the eyes that can be seen on the retina of the eyes. Diabetes causes a weakening of the tiny blood vessels in the eyes, and they may eventually rupture and form retinal hemorrhages. These hemorrhages can form clots that may eventually cause retinal detachment.

- If you are diabetic, it is very important that an ophthalmologist examines you annually. An ophthalmologist will examine the eyes, thoroughly checking for signs of retinopathy. He may decide to use laser surgery to save your vision, but as a result of laser surgery, some may have minor loss of vision as well as a decrease in night vision. This is why it is critically important to maintain good blood sugar control if diabetic retinopathy is detected.

- *Kidney disease.* In the United States, diabetes is the underlying cause of approximately half of the people who require long-term dialysis, as well as being the leading cause of kidney failure.[16]

- However, don't let these statistics scare you. The majority of people with diabetes do *not* develop kidney disease, and of those who do, most do not progress to kidney failure. This is good news. It means that even with diabetes, simply controlling your blood sugar will almost always prevent kidney disease.

- Controlling your blood sugar and blood pressure, along with maintaining a healthy diet and losing weight, is critically important if you are facing the challenge of kidney disease. Your doctor may prescribe a medication such as an ACE inhibitor, and I recommend a form of vitamin B_6, which also helps to protect the kidneys. You will learn more about this in chapter 5.

- Kidney failure can be avoided if kidney disease is detected early on. But the early stages of kidney disease usually remain undetected with a regular urinalysis. Therefore, it's important to get a specific test for microalbumin that can detect protein in the urine years before a regular urinalysis can. Make sure your doctor checks the microalbumin level in your urine annually at least.

- *Diabetic neuropathy.* Long-term diabetes eventually affects the nerves, leading to diabetic neuropathy. Approximately 60 to 70 percent of diabetics have some form of peripheral nerve damage, which often affects the feet and hands, and the patient usually describes symptoms of numbness or decreased ability to feel light touch and pain.[17] They also usually develop burning and tingling or extreme sensitivity to touch, especially in their feet, and their symptoms are usually worse at night.

- Diabetic neuropathy may eventually lead to foot ulcers. Sometimes these foot ulcers become infected, and if not treated promptly, they may lead to severe infection and eventual amputation. Maintaining good foot care, wearing comfortable shoes and socks, carefully inspecting your feet daily, and maintaining good blood sugar control are very important in treating diabetic neuropathy. Also, I recommend to my diabetic patients to never go outdoors barefoot.

- I also recommend that people with diabetic neuropathy see a podiatrist or foot specialist on a regular basis. In chapter 5, you will find great nutritional supplements that are usually very effective in helping diabetic neuropathy.

- *Amputations.* More than half of lower-limb amputations in the United States occur among people with diabetes. In recent years, this number has been as high as seventy-one thousand lower-limb amputations per year being performed on people with diabetes.[18] The lower extremities are more susceptible to the circulatory impairment caused by diabetes simply because they are further from the heart. The nutrients and oxygen in the bloodstream must make their way through a much greater distance of blood vessels and capillaries to nourish cells in the feet and toes.

- *Dental disease.* Dental disease, in the form of periodontal disease (a type of gum disease that can lead to tooth loss), occurs with greater frequency and severity among people with diabetes. People with poorly controlled diabetes are three times more likely to develop severe periodontitis than those without diabetes.[19]

- *Pregnancy complications.* Poorly controlled diabetes prior to conception and during the first three months of pregnancy can cause major birth defects and even spontaneous abortion. During the second and third trimesters, if diabetes is not controlled, it can result in large babies, posing a risk to both mother and child.[20]

- *Other illnesses.* Diabetics are also more susceptible to other illnesses and have a worse prognosis if they do come down with these illnesses. For instance, diabetics are more likely to die from flu and pneumonia than nondiabetics.[21]

- *Erectile dysfunction.* A very common complication of diabetes is impotence or erectile dysfunction, which is the inability to have or sustain an erection sufficient for intercourse. It is estimated that 50 to 60 percent of diabetic men over the age of fifty will experience erectile dysfunction.[22] However, if discovered early enough, this can be prevented or even reversed by losing belly fat, controlling blood sugar with diet and exercise, stress reduction, and taking supplements and hormone replacement.

THE GOOD NEWS

After reading through all of these dismal complications, you may feel like tiny David when he stood before the nine-foot giant called Goliath. Don't give in to fear. These are the complications that most often affect diabetics whose blood sugar levels are not controlled through proper diet and exercise.

In the face of these medical facts, your goal is to take advantage of the wealth of wisdom in God's Word and in the medical knowledge He has given us over the centuries to avoid these complications altogether by making wise choices. Most importantly, your primary goal is to take hold of the healing Jesus offers you.

A **BIBLE** **CURE** *Prayer for You*

Dear heavenly Father, help me make wise choices and follow the guidelines in Your Word concerning food choices, lifestyle, prayer, and a thought life that is saturated with Your living Word. Thank You for hearing and answering my prayer so I will be free to serve You with my whole mind, body, soul, and strength. Amen.

But he was pierced for our rebellion, crushed for our sins. He was beaten so we could be whole. He was whipped so we could be healed.

—ISAIAH 53:5

Write out this verse, and insert your own name into it: "He was pierced for _____'s rebellion, He was crushed for _____'s sins; He was beaten so that _____ could be made whole and whipped so that _____ could be healed!"

Write out a personal prayer to Jesus Christ, thanking Him for exchanging His health for your pain. Thank Him for taking the power of sickness onto His own body so that He could purchase your healing from diabetes.

_____

_____

_____

_____

_____

_____

_____

_____

2

BATTLE DIABETES WITH GOOD NUTRITION

THE SAME GOD who skillfully designed your body as an incredible, living creation and created your pancreas to produce insulin also designed the human body to operate at peak efficiency and health when it is supplied with proper nutrition. If you are a diabetic, what you eat makes all the difference in the world!

Ask God to give you a new way of looking at nutrition. You'll be surprised at the way your thinking about food begins to change. First, and most importantly, you must stop looking at the scale and start looking at your waistline as a key indicator of weight management.

YOUR WAISTLINE IS YOUR LIFELINE

Why wait until you have a major complication like the list we covered at the end of chapter 1 before you start controlling your blood sugar? Take a proactive approach to diabetes by first realizing that your waistline is your lifeline. If your waist measurement increases, your blood sugar will typically increase, and if your waist measurement decreases, your blood sugar will typically decrease. By focusing on your waistline and following a doctor's plan and exercise advice to shrink your waist, you will find that your blood sugar will lower according to your waist measurement.

Let's start with an understanding of how to measure your waist. Over the years, I've discovered that many men do not measure their waists correctly. They may have a 52-inch waist, but they don't realize it because they still fit into jeans with a 32-inch waist. Their huge bellies are hanging over their belts, and yet they are adamant that they have a 32-inch waist.

Also, over the last several years, low-waisted pants have become popular in many women's clothing styles. As a result, I have seen more and more women measuring too low for their waist measurement as well.

Your waist is measured around your belly button (and around your love handles if you have them). I have had patients who were shocked by the reality of their true waist measurement once I showed them the proper place to measure. As the reality sinks in, I help them devise the following plan to reach their waist measurement goal.

First, put away your scale since daily or weekly weighing usually leads to disappointment, and you may eventually give up. Instead, follow your waist measurement on a monthly basis.

Second, establish a waist measurement goal. Initially, the waist measurement goal for a man with diabetes or prediabetes is 40 inches or less. For a woman with prediabetes or diabetes the goal is to have a waist measurement of 35 inches or less.

Third, take your height in inches and divide it by two. Eventually, your waist measurement should be equal to this number or less. In other words, your waist should measure half of your height or less. For example, a 5-foot-8-inch man would be 68 inches tall, so his waist should be 34 inches or less around the belly button and love handles.

Notice that this is the *third* step, especially for prediabetics and type 2 diabetics. Decrease your waist to 40 inches or less (for men) or 35 inches or less (for women) before you worry about getting it down to half your height or less.

I can promise you that you will be amazed as your blood sugar drops with every inch lost in your waist.

WHAT IS THE GLYCEMIC INDEX?

The glycemic index gives an indication of the rate at which different carbs break down to release sugar into the bloodstream. More precisely, it assesses a numeric value to how rapidly the blood sugar rises after consuming a food that contains carbohydrates. Keep in mind the fact that the glycemic index is only for carbohydrates and not for fats or proteins.

Sugars and carbohydrates that are digested rapidly, such as white bread, white rice, and instant potatoes, raise the blood sugar rapidly. These are considered high-glycemic foods because they have a glycemic index of 70 or higher. If the glycemic index for a certain food is high, then it will raise your blood sugar levels much faster (this is bad). High blood sugar levels, in turn, increase the amount of insulin that will be secreted by type 2 diabetics and prediabetics to bring the blood sugar level back into balance.

> Don't worry about anything; instead, pray about
> everything. Tell God what you need, and thank him
> for all he has done. Then you will experience God's
> peace, which exceeds anything we can understand.
> His peace will guard your hearts and minds as you
> live in Christ Jesus.
>
> —PHILIPPIANS 4:6–7

On the other hand, if foods containing carbohydrates are digested slowly and therefore release sugars gradually or slowly into the bloodstream, they have a low glycemic index value of 55 or lower. These foods include most vegetables and fruits, beans, peas, lentils, sweet potatoes, and the like. Because these foods cause the blood sugar to rise more slowly, insulin levels do not rise significantly and the blood sugar levels are stabilized for a longer period of time. Low-glycemic foods also cause satiety hormones to be released in the small intestines, which keeps you satisfied longer.

As an example of the various glycemic index values for different foods, glucose has a value of 100, while broccoli and cabbage, both of which contain little or no carbohydrates, have a value of 0 to 1. In truth, there is nothing fancy about the glycemic index. One of the most important factors that can determine the food's glycemic index value is simply how much the food has been processed. Generally speaking, the more highly processed a food, the higher its glycemic index value; the more natural a food, the lower its glycemic index value.

A **BIBLE CURE** *Health Tip*
Rule of Thumb: The Glycemic Index
Low-glycemic foods are 55 or less.
Medium-glycemic foods are 56 to 69.
High-glycemic foods are 70 and above.

THE GLYCEMIC LOAD

Almost twenty years after the glycemic index was established as a standard of measurement, researchers at Harvard University developed a new way of classifying foods that took into account not only the glycemic index value of a food but also the quantity of carbohydrates that food contains. This is called the glycemic load (GL). It gives us a guide as to how much quantity of a particular carbohydrate or food we should eat.

For a while, nutritionists scratched their heads as patients desiring to lose weight were eating low-glycemic foods yet were not losing weight. In fact, some were actually gaining weight. The problem, they discovered through the GL, was that over-consuming many types of low-glycemic foods can actually lead to weight gain. And these patients were eating as many low-glycemic foods as they wanted, simply because they had been told that foods with a low glycemic index value were better for weight loss.

You can determine the glycemic load of a food by multiplying the glycemic index value by the quantity of carbohydrates a serving contains (in grams), and then dividing that number by 100. The actual formula looks like this:

(Glycemic index value x *carb grams per serving)* / 100 = *glycemic load*

To show you how important the GL is, let me offer some examples. Some wheat pastas have a low glycemic index value, which makes many dieters think they're an automatic key to losing weight. However, if a serving size of that wheat pasta is too large, it may sabotage your weight loss efforts because, despite a low glycemic index value, the GL is high. On the other extreme, watermelon has a high glycemic index value but a very low GL, which makes it OK to eat in a larger quantity. Yet another example, the GL of white potatoes is double that of sweet potatoes.

> You must serve only the LORD your God. If you do, I will bless you with food and water, and I will protect you from illness.
>
> —EXODUS 23:25

Don't worry, I am not recommending that you calculate the GL for every item at every meal you eat. The main point is that by understanding the GL, you can identify which low-glycemic foods can cause trouble if you eat too much of them. These include low-glycemic breads, low-glycemic rice, sweet potatoes, low-glycemic pasta, and low-glycemic cereals. As a general rule, any large quantity of a low-glycemic "starchy" food will usually have a high GL, so limit the serving to no larger than a tennis ball.

Keep in mind also that if you use the GL without considering the glycemic index, you will probably be eating more of an Atkins-type diet with lots of fats and proteins and very few carbohydrates—which is not a healthy way to eat in the long run and can cause insulin resistance.

A BIBLE CURE *Health Tip*

Glycemic Index Values of Common Foods[1]

To look up the glycemic index values of other foods not listed here, go to www.glycemicindex.com.

Food	Glycemic Index Value
Asparagus	<15
Broccoli	<15
Celery	<15
Cucumber	<15
Green beans	<15
Lettuce (all varieties)	<15
Low-fat yogurt (artificially sweetened)	<15
Peppers (all varieties)	<15
Spinach	<15
Zucchini	<15
Tomatoes	15
Cherries	22
Milk (skim)	32
Spaghetti (whole wheat)	37
Apples	38
All-Bran cereal	42
Lentil soup (tinned)	44
Whole-grain bread	50

Food	Glycemic Index Value
Orange juice	52
Bananas	54
Potato (sweet)	54
Rice (brown)	55
Popcorn	55
Muesli	56
Whole-meal bread	69
Watermelon	72
Doughnut	76
Rice cakes	77
Corn Flakes	83
Potato (baked)	85
Baguette	95
Parsnips	97
Dates	103

Additional foods with high glycemic index levels that you need to limit or avoid include instant potatoes, instant rice, French bread, white bread, corn, processed oats, instant potatoes, white rice, most boxed cereals (such as cornflakes), baked potatoes, mashed potatoes, cooked carrots, honey, raisins, dried fruit, candy bars, crackers, cookies, ice cream, and pastries. If you are diabetic, you should either eat these foods very rarely or avoid them completely.

Remember that high-glycemic foods and high-density carbohydrates raise blood sugar quickly, which in turn raises insulin levels. When this occurs long term, the high insulin levels cause your cells to become resistant to insulin. You might say that these high-glycemic foods are similar to a toxin in an individual with type 2 diabetes.

> If you will listen carefully to the voice of the LORD your God and do what is right in his sight, obeying his commands and keeping all his decrees, then I will not make you suffer any of the diseases I sent on the Egyptians; for I am the LORD who heals you.
>
> —EXODUS 15:26

If you are dealing with type 2 diabetes, your pancreas may be producing about four times as much insulin as a nondiabetic's pancreas. The key to correcting your cells' resistance to insulin is following the proper diet. You must decrease or avoid sugars and high-glycemic starches, such as breads, white rice, potatoes, and corn, and decrease fats, including saturated fats, and fried foods. If you will do this, your cells will eventually recover. They will begin to regain their sensitivity to insulin. You hold the key.

THE BIBLE AND FATS

Interestingly, eating certain fats is condemned in the Bible. God commands, "You must never eat any fat or blood. This is a permanent law for you, and it must be observed from generation to generation, wherever you live" (Lev. 3:17). This verse is referring to the toxic belly fat of the animal, which also includes the fat around the kidneys and liver. The fat in this verse is also translated "grease." God created our bodies and knows how they have been designed to function best. I encourage you to substitute a small amount of extra-virgin olive oil and flaxseed oil as well as other healthy oils for butter, cream, and other fats. Do not cook with flaxseed oil. Always choose low-fat portions of meat as well. Especially avoid trans fats, hydrogenated fats, and partially hydrogenated fats. Excessive amounts of saturated fats and any trans fats are associated with insulin resistance. For more information on this topic, refer to *The Seven Pillars of Health*.

A **BIBLE CURE** Health Tip
Antidiabetogenic Foods

Gabriel Cousens, MD, author of *There Is a Cure for Diabetes*, recommends the following foods for their therapeutic properties in the treatment of diabetes.[2]

- Jerusalem artichoke—an herbal medicine that contains inulin, which prevents your blood sugar from rising rapidly.

- Bitter melon—a green tropical fruit that resembles a cucumber and contains several antidiabetic properties.

- Cucumber—contains a hormone your pancreas needs to produce insulin.

- Celery—has general antidiabetogenic qualities and also helps lower your blood pressure, which is a symptom of metabolic syndrome.

- Garlic and onion—contain sulfur compounds believed to be the reason for their antidiabetic effects.

- Walnuts—a handful contains high amounts of monounsaturated fat, omega-3 fatty acid, and alpha linolenic acid (ALA), which help to lower cholesterol and fats in your blood and are important in protecting against diabetes.
- Almonds—a handful provides vitamin E, magnesium, and fiber. The *Journal of Nutrition* reported that almonds and walnuts provide glycemic control when you add them to a high-carbohydrate meal.
- Kelp—this sea vegetable promotes thyroid health, and your thyroid controls your metabolism, which in turn affects your ability to lose weight.

FANTASTIC FIBER

Another important way you can battle diabetes through nutrition is to increase the fiber in your diet. Dietary fiber is extremely important in helping to control diabetes. Fiber slows down digestion and the absorption of carbohydrates. This allows for a more gradual rise in blood sugar.

If you have diabetes, a significant amount of the carbohydrate calories you eat should come from vegetables, including peas, beans, lentils, and legumes. Those vegetables typically contain large amounts of fiber. The more soluble fiber in your diet, the better blood sugar control your body will have.

> That is why I tell you not to worry about everyday life—whether you have enough food and drink, or enough clothes to wear. Isn't life more than food, and your body more than clothing? Look at the birds. They don't plant or harvest or store food in barns, for your heavenly Father feeds them. And aren't you far more valuable to him than they are?
>
> —MATTHEW 6:25–26

Water-soluble fibers are found in oat bran, seeds such as psyllium (the primary ingredient in Metamucil), fruit and vegetables (especially apples and pears), beans, and nuts. You should try to take in at least 30 to 35 g of fiber a day. You also should take the fiber with meals in order to prevent rapid rises in blood sugar.

A BIBLE CURE Health Tip
Increasing Fiber in Your Diet

You might try the following ideas to increase the fiber in your diet:

1. Eat at least five servings of fruit and vegetables each day. Fruit and vegetables that are high in fiber include:

- Granny Smith apples
- Peas
- Broccoli
- Spinach
- Berries
- Pears
- Brussels sprouts
- Beans (all types)
- Parsnips
- Legumes
- Carrots (not cooked)
- Lentils

2. Replace breads and cereals made from refined flours with whole-grain breads and cereals. Eat brown rice instead of white rice. Examples of these foods include:

- Walnuts, almonds, and macadamia nuts
- Old-fashioned steel-cut oatmeal or high-fiber instant oatmeal
- Brown rice
- Flaxseeds, chia seeds, hemp seeds, pumpkin seeds, and sunflower seeds
- Ezekiel bread or other sprouted bread

3. Eat high-fiber cereal for breakfast. Check labels on the packages for the amounts of dietary fiber in each brand. Some cereals may have less fiber than you think. Fiber One cereal, Kashi Cinnamon Harvest, and Kashi Island Vanilla are good choices

4. Eat cooked beans, peas, or lentils a few times a week.

5. Take PGX fiber (two to three capsules with 16 oz. of water before each meal.

Many foods contain dietary fiber. Eating foods that are high in fiber can not only help relieve some problems with diabetes but also may help lower your cholesterol and even prevent heart disease and certain types of cancer.

A WORD OF CAUTION

When adding fiber to your diet, make small changes over a period of time to help prevent bloating, cramping, or gas. Start by adding one of the items listed above to your diet, then wait several days or even a week before making another change. If one change doesn't seem to work for you, try a different one.

It's important to drink more fluids when you increase the amount of fiber you eat. Drink at least two additional glasses of water a day when you increase your fiber intake.

This information provides a general overview on dietary fiber and may not apply to everyone. I have included some advice in chapter 4 and chapter 5 to help you increase your fiber intake through diet and nutritional supplements. I also recommend reading my book *Dr. Colbert's "I Can Do This" Diet*.

A BIBLE CURE Health Tip
Avoid Soy

For the last few years I have been warning people about the use of soy because I've seen many people have adverse reactions to consuming it. Others in the medical community are beginning to speak out as well.

Gabriel Cousens, MD, calls soy a *diabetogenic* food, meaning it produces diabetes. Cousens explains that 90 percent of all soy is genetically modified (GMO). Soy is also one of the top seven allergens. The isoflavones in soy can make a person estrogenic, contributing to cancer of the breast, and uterine fibroids. Cousens also links soy to decreased thyroid production, stunted growth in children, lowering of good (HDL) cholesterol, insulin resistance, heart disease, and Alzheimer's disease.[3]

WHAT ABOUT BREAD?

Americans love white bread, coffee, and hot dogs. However, processing white bread removes all the bran and germ, along with approximately 80 percent of the nutrients and virtually all the fiber. Bleaching the flour destroys even more vitamins. Sugar and hydrogenated fats are added, right along with manufactured vitamins. In the end you get a product that is pure starch—stripped of the fiber and nutritional value of whole-grain breads. Add water to white bread, and it forms a sticky, glue-like substance. Is there any wonder why this food takes double the amount of time to be eliminated from the body?

America's romance with processed foods, such as breads, potatoes, and other grains, is one of the main reasons we see diabetes increasing every year at alarming rates.

> I know how to live on almost nothing or with everything. I have learned the secret of living in every situation, whether it is with a full stomach or empty, with plenty or little. For I can do everything through Christ, who gives me strength.
> —PHILIPPIANS 4:12–13

Today the best choices of bread are the sprouted breads found in most health food stores. I personally choose Ezekiel bread, which is made of the sprouts of wheat, barley, and other grains.

Remember, even if breads at the supermarket are called whole-grain breads, they also may contain sugar and hydrogenated fats and are processed in such a way that they still have fairly high glycemic indexes. Therefore, if my diabetic patients request bread, I recommend that they have moderate amounts of sprouted bread, such as Ezekiel bread, in the morning or at lunch. I find that it tastes better when toasted. You can find Ezekiel bread in many grocery stores in the frozen food section and online. Try it. You'll love the taste! The new double-fiber breads are a step in the right direction, but I still prefer the sprouted breads.

A BIBLE CURE *Health Fact*
Coffee Lowers Risk of Developing Diabetes

Three different studies have shown that coffee consumption helps decrease the risk of developing type 2 diabetes. An analysis of over seventeen thousand Dutch men and women found that the more coffee a person drinks, the lower the risk for developing type 2 diabetes. Consuming three to four cups of coffee a day decreased the risk of developing diabetes by 23 percent, and people who drank over seven cups a day cut their risk in half.[4]

A Finnish study found that consuming three to four cups of coffee a day decreased type 2 diabetes risk by 24 percent, and consuming ten or more cups a day lowered the risk by 61 percent.[5]

Another study of coffee consumption explored the benefits of caffeinated versus decaffeinated coffee. Men who drank one to three cups of decaf coffee a day decreased their risk of diabetes by 9 percent while those who drank four or more cups a day lowered it by 26 percent.[6]

Please note that these studies pertain to *preventing* diabetes. More studies are needed before we can conclusively state the effects of coffee in people who are already diabetic. Some studies have shown that excessive caffeine raises blood sugar, and unfortunately, most Americans consume their coffee loaded with sugar and cream that are likely to raise blood sugar as well. For this reason, I do not advise people with diabetes to drink more than one or two cups of organic coffee (sweetened with stevia) per day.

If you are interested in preventing diabetes, an alternative to drinking coffee is taking coffee berry extract. Coffee berry is the fruit that produces coffee beans. The powerful phytonutrients that quench free radicals and help manage blood sugar are found in the whole fruit and not just the bean. I generally recommend 100 mg of coffee berry extract, three times a day.

A FINAL WORD

In summary, proper diet is still the cornerstone for treating diabetes. If you are a type 1 diabetic, you must avoid sugar altogether and dramatically limit starches. Limit fruit as well, because it can also raise your blood sugar dramatically. High-fiber foods such as legumes (beans) and root vegetables (uncooked carrots) will help to lower your blood sugar. Type 1 diabetics must also avoid fruit juices. Your physician or dietician should closely monitor your diet.

However, if you are a type 2 diabetic, you can benefit from small amounts of low-glycemic fruit that is high in fiber, such as pears and Granny Smith apples, if they are used conservatively. Do not drink fruit juice or eat applesauce.

The most important dietary advice is to avoid sugar and to dramatically limit refined starches, including white breads, refined pasta, potatoes, most cereals, white rice, and other highly processed foods.

A **BIBLE CURE** Prayer for You

Dear heavenly Father, You are the One who will help me throughout my life if I let You. You don't expect me to be perfect, just to receive You into my life. When I've blown it in the way I eat and the way I live, You are ready to forgive and help me to stay on course. Your power to forgive is as great as Your power to love. I will never forget how much You love me. Amen.

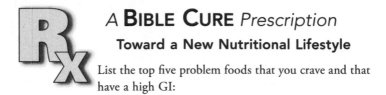

A **BIBLE CURE** *Prescription*
Toward a New Nutritional Lifestyle

List the top five problem foods that you crave and that have a high GI:

_____

_____

_____

_____

_____

List five healthy food choices you will make this week instead:

_____

_____

_____

_____

_____

In what ways do you need God's help to change your eating habits?

_____

_____

_____

_____

_____

Write out a Bible cure prayer asking for God's help in making these changes.

_____

_____

_____

_____

_____

BATTLE DIABETES WITH ACTIVITY

Your body, the dwelling place of God's Spirit, needs to be protected and kept healthy. Remember, your body was bought by the blood of Jesus, and you are to glorify God in your body and in your spirit (1 Cor. 6:20). You must do your part, which involves choosing the correct foods and beverages and exercising the body on a regular basis. You must take courage and continually battle diabetes because it can weaken and damage other organs in your body.

I cannot stress enough how important it is to overcome your diabetes with exercise. Exercise holds special benefits for diabetics. Multiple studies have shown that those who have a physically active lifestyle are less prone to develop type 2 diabetes. I believe this is because physical exercise battles the root of type 2 diabetes, which gets its start when muscle cells lose their sensitivity to insulin. Research has shown that your muscle cells are much less likely to become resistant to insulin if you keep them fit through regular exercise.

Studies have also shown that regular exercise improves glucose tolerance and lowers blood sugar as well as insulin requirements. The more muscle tissue that we develop in our large muscle groups such as the thighs and buttocks, the more sugar will be removed from the bloodstream. The greater the muscle mass in especially the large muscle groups is likey associated with a corresponding drop in insulin resistance. Also, by burning calories, exercise helps control weight, an important factor in the management of type 2 diabetes.

A study at the Cooper Institute for Aerobics Research in Dallas shows that staying fit may be the most important thing you can do to avoid type 2 diabetes. The researchers put 8,633 men with an average age of forty-three through a treadmill test and then screened them for diabetes six years later. The men who scored poorly on the fitness test were almost four times more likely to have developed the disease than those who had done well on the treadmill. In fact, the fitness scores turned out to be the most accurate predictor of diabetes—more than age, obesity, high blood pressure, or family history of the disease.[1]

A **BIBLE CURE** Health Tip
Important!

Before undergoing any activity or fitness program, please check with your doctor to make sure that you are healthy enough to participate.

If you don't participate in at least thirty minutes of exercise per day, talk with your doctor about ways to incorporate more exercise into your everyday life. Because I'm a doctor and have advised many patients over the years, I know that most people immediately visualize exercise as just another chore, or they think it will be embarrassing, draining, or very unpleasant. So instead of exercise, let's simply think of this as "increasing your activity level." Here are a few quick tips to get you started:

- First, you need to choose an activity that is fun and enjoyable. You will never stick to any activity program if you dread or hate it.
- Also, I find it is best to do your activity program with a friend or partner.
- Make sure that you wear comfortable, well-fitting shoes and socks.
- If you are a type 1 diabetic, you will need to work with your doctor in order to adjust your insulin doses while increasing your activity. Realize that exercising will lower your blood sugar; this can be potentially dangerous in a type 1 diabetic.

Now, let's discuss the different types of activities you can choose from.

AEROBIC ACTIVITY

Examples of aerobic activity are walking, cycling, swimming, working out on an elliptical machine, dancing, and hiking; it's any movement that raises the heart rate enough to help you burn fat. I used to have patients figure out their training heart rate zone and keep their heart rate in that zone. This is certainly good to do, and with new aerobic exercise equipment, one simply holds onto the handles and the machine calculates your heart rate for you. However, I've found that most diabetics hate going to a gym and simply will not exercise. For them, I recommend the perceived exertion scale.

A **BIBLE CURE** *Health Tip*
Perceived Exertion Scale

This is a scale that ranks your perceived exertion as:

1. Very, very light
2. Very light
3. Fairly light
4. Somewhat hard
5. Very hard
6. Very, very hard

Usually, when you exercise at a perceived exertion of somewhat hard, you are typically in your target heart rate zone.

One of the best aerobic activities is simply brisk walking. A very simple way to enter your target heart rate zone is to simply walk briskly enough so that you cannot sing and slowly enough so that you can talk. This simple formula works for most of my patients. If you are walking so slow that you can sing, simply speed up. But if you are walking so fast that you cannot talk, then slow down. This is another reason why you need an activity partner or buddy to talk with as you walk.

For diabetic patients with foot ulcers or numbness in the feet, walking is not the best activity for you. Instead, try cycling, the elliptical machine, or pool activities. Be sure to inspect your feet well before and after your activity session.

If you are able to walk, simply walk in your neighborhood or a nearby park, starting with a five- or ten-minute walk, and increase it gradually as tolerated. Many of my patients eventually prefer to walk for ten to fifteen minutes in the morning after breakfast and ten to fifteen minutes in the evening after dinner.

By breaking up the activity program into two shorter time segments, most people find it easier to handle. Simply walking your dog twice a day will usually do the trick. It is also good to walk as a family after dinner and use the time to connect with each other, laugh, and unwind.

RESISTANCE EXERCISES

Resistance training usually involves lifting weights to build muscles. I have shared this simple rule of thumb with my diabetic patients for years: the more muscle you build in the lower extremities and buttocks, generally the better blood sugar control you will have.

> While dining with a ruler, pay attention to what is put before you. If you are a big eater, put a knife to your throat; don't desire all the delicacies, for he might be trying to trick you.
>
> —PROVERBS 23:1–3

Scientific studies have proven that a combination of resistance training and aerobic exercise is the most effective way to improve insulin sensitivities in diabetics.[2] That is why I call aerobic activity and resistance training a one-two punch to knock out type 2 diabetes.

Aerobic activity combined with resistance training will

improve blood sugar control even better than most diabetic medications.

I usually start patients with simple resistance exercises like those I describe in my book *The Seven Pillars of Health* and eventually graduate them to resistance exercises with weights. I strongly recommend starting with a certified personal trainer in order to instruct you in the proper technique and to develop a good resistance program with emphasis on increasing strength and muscle mass in the lower extremities.

Over time, I find that most diabetics benefit from activity five days a week, with at least thirty to forty-five minutes of aerobic activity and fifteen to thirty minutes of resistance exercises three times a week. Remember, this one-two punch of resistance training and aerobic activity is better than medication for diabetes.

STICKING WITH IT

Many people find that, difficult as it is to start an exercise program, it is even more difficult to stick with it. Too many people get into trouble when they save exercising for their spare time. If you wait until you can get around to it, you probably never will. Make exercise a priority as important as a doctor's appointment.

> Do you like honey? Don't eat too much, or it will make you sick! . . . It's not good to eat too much honey.
> —PROVERBS 25:16, 27

Choose an exercise activity that you truly enjoy. Walking is only one suggestion. Have you tried ballroom dancing? Or backpacking? Perhaps you've always pictured yourself on a tennis court. Surely there is an activity that you always thought you'd like to try. Now's the time—try it. If you enjoy it, then stick with it.

In addition, most people feel calm and have a sense of well-being after they exercise. You can actually walk off your anxieties. Exercise releases endorphins, which are morphine-like substances that give us feelings of well-being. People who exercise feel better about themselves, look better, feel more energetic, and are more productive at work.

NOW, TAKE THE OFFENSIVE!

Take the offensive, and follow the positive steps suggested in this chapter. You will discover how effective God's wisdom can be in both the spiritual and natural realms. God heals in many ways, whether through supernatural means or through the more gradual—but equally divine—means of proper nutrition, exercise, and biblical life choices.

A BIBLE CURE Prayer for You

Lord, help me to change my habits. I need Your strength and determination when mine weakens. Give me the desire and motivation I need to succeed. Lord Jesus, I choose to believe that the power of the cross is greater than my bondage to diabetes. You love me and died on the cross to free me from all of my bondages. I crucify my flesh daily and choose to give it what it needs and not what it craves. I now know it needs exercise and increased activity. I, (your name), *choose faith today,* (date). *I give You these* (how many pounds) *pounds—and confess by faith that I weigh* _____ *pounds* (define goal). *In Jesus's name I declare victory today! Amen.*

A **Bible Cure** *Prescription*

Battling Diabetes With Exercise

What activity or exercise are you getting at least five days a week?

_____

_____

_____

_____

How are you monitoring your heart rate?

_____

_____

_____

_____

What are your goals for increasing the amount of activity or exercise you get regularly?

_____

_____

_____

_____

Think about what partner you will choose to be your exercise buddy—your neighbor, friend, spouse, child, etc.

_____

_____

_____

_____

What time is best to make in your schedule to have a consistent exercise time? Your exercise time should be viewed as important as a doctor's appointment.

_____

_____

_____

_____

_____

_____

_____

BATTLE DIABETES WITH WEIGHT LOSS

H AVE YOU BEEN battling a weight problem all of your life with little or no success? No one has to tell you that many cases of diabetes are directly linked to obesity. Determine right now that, with God's help, you will get to your ideal weight and stay there. Perhaps you've been overweight for so long that you've given up. In the back of your mind you may even be thinking, "It's impossible for me to lose weight."

The Bible says, "Nothing is impossible with God" (Luke 1:37). It may seem virtually impossible for you alone. But you are not alone! God is on your side, and His strength is available to help you.

Don't even try to face this issue alone. You don't have to. At this moment, whisper a prayer with me asking God to strengthen you to overcome any sense of defeat and bondage that obesity has caused in your life.

A POWERFUL KEY TO PREVENTION

Weight control is a powerful key to the reversal and the prevention of diabetes. Type 2 diabetes is directly linked to obesity and diets rich in sugars, refined carbohydrates, and fats. Since it is far better to prevent diabetes altogether rather than to reverse the disease and ask God to heal you afterward, I strongly encourage you to lose weight if necessary if you are seeking to prevent diabetes. If you already have type 2 diabetes, weight control is absolutely essential.

YOUR IDEAL WEIGHT—CATCH THE VISION!

Close your eyes, and picture yourself walking around in the body that God intended for you to have—the healthy one. You don't have to shop in plus-size stores anymore. You move easily and confidently and no longer huff and puff when you climb stairs. You will wear a bathing suit with comfort and confidence. Are you catching the vision?

It is absolutely essential that you see yourself weighing a healthy weight on a daily basis and place a picture of yourself at a healthy weight around the house, on your vanity mirror, or on your fridge. Then confess daily that you weigh your desired weight by faith.

As you visualize yourself weighting a certain weight or being a certain size and confess it daily, you reset your mental auto-pilot, and you will start to lose weight. Do not say, "I will lose 30 or 40 pounds by faith," or else you will always have 30 or 40 pounds to lose.

So whether you eat or drink, or whatever you do, do it all for the glory of God.

—1 CORINTHIANS 10:31

Write down your desired weight in the space provided.

My desired weight is _____ pounds.
My actual weight is _____ pounds.
I need to lose _____ pounds.

Realize that your waist measurement is more important than your weight. Remember, your eventual goal is a waist measurement of less than half of your height.

A **BIBLE CURE** *Health Fact*

BMI, Waist Size, and Type 2 Diabetes

Various health organizations, including the Centers for Disease Control and Prevention (CDC) and the National Institutes of Health (NIH), officially define the terms *overweight* and *obesity* using the body mass index (BMI), which factors in a person's weight relative to height. Most of these organizations define an overweight adult as having a BMI between 25 and 29.9, while an obese adult is anyone who has a BMI of 30 or higher.[1] If you would like a chart to help you determine your BMI, refer to my book *The Seven Pillars of Health* or conduct an online search for "BMI" and take advantage of the many Web sites with tools to help you calculate your BMI.

However, I believe an even more important measurement to focus on is your waist size. The larger your waist, the greater your chances of having type 2 diabetes. In fact, it's been proven that, for men, waist size is an even better predictor of diabetes than BMI. A thirteen-year study of more than twenty-seven thousand men discovered that:

- A waist size of 34 to 36 doubled diabetes risk.
- A waist size of 36 to 38 nearly tripled the risk.
- A waist size of 38 to 40 was associated with five times the risk.
- A waist size of 40 to 62 was associated with twelve times the risk.[2]

DR. COLBERT'S RAPID WAIST REDUCTION DIET

This Bible cure combines faith in God with practical steps, as you know by now. So, here is the practical side: the diet. I recommend you use the rules of good nutrition for diabetics outlined in chapter 2 on nutrition and create a daily diet using my Rapid Waist Reduction Diet. The key is to eat no complex carbs after 6:00 p.m. other than beans or lentils. Make sure to choose the *organic* form of any of the allowable foods listed below.

Allowable foods

Breakfast

- Two to three free-range or organic eggs, omega-3 egg yolk, three egg whites per day, or one scoop of Life's Basics Plant Protein (see appendix) with 8 oz. of coconut milk, coconut kefir (from a health food store), skim milk, or low-fat plain kefir

- Two- to three-egg omelet with plenty of veggies (onions, avocado, tomatoes, etc.); use one whole egg or three egg whites

- ½ cup steel-cut oatmeal (tennis ball–sized serving) or the new high-fiber instant oatmeal (if time is a factor)
- 1 Tbsp. almonds, walnuts, or pecans
- ½ cup berries, one Granny Smith apple, or one pear

Lunch

- As much salad as you want. Salads may include any of the following: avocado, celery, chives, cilantro, cucumber, greens, parsley, red or yellow peppers, sprouts, and tomatoes.
- A sweet potato the size of a tennis ball, or ½ cup beans, peas, or lentils
- Homemade salad dressings in a salad spritzer (dressing can be made using four parts vinegar to one part extra-virgin olive oil and may include garlic, lime, lemon, and cilantro), or you may use salad spritzers such as Ken's or Wishbone
- 1 Tbsp. of seeds or nuts (1 Tbsp. = about ten nuts), or 1 Tbsp. of any of the following oils: grape seed oil mayonnaise, extra-virgin olive oil, coconut butter, organic butter (check labels to make sure you choose oils that are non GMO)
- Vegetable or bean soup (non-cream-based soups)
- 3–4 oz. for females or 4–5 oz. for males of lean protein (chicken, turkey, tongol tuna, salmon, sardines, extra-lean red meat, etc.) grilled, baked,

or broiled, not fried (limit red meat to 18 oz. or less a week)

Dinner

- 3–5 oz. of protein (allowable sources of protein are lean meats, poultry, eggs, and fish such as wild Alaskan salmon, tongol tuna, and sardines)
- As many steamed, stir-fried, grilled, or raw vegetables as you want. Allowable veggies are asparagus, bok choy, broccoli, brussels sprouts, cabbage, cauliflower, celery, chard, Chinese cabbage, eggplant, green beans, green chilies, kale, leeks, onions, snow peas, sprouts, tomatoes, and zucchini. Many foods from Thailand typically (or Thai restaurants) contain these veggies.
- Fresh herbs and spices to flavor foods to taste
- Salad and salad dressing, as described on the previous page
- ½ cup legumes and beans, peas, or lentils (tennis ball–sized serving); bean soup; or hummus

Beverages

- Lemonade or limeade made from fresh lemon or lime with water, sweetened with stevia
- Green, white, or black tea sweetened with stevia

Foods to limit or avoid

- Dairy: if you must eat dairy, eat it for breakfast, and limit it to skim or 1 percent organic milk or organic, plain, low-fat kefir and yogurt (I prefer coconut kefir)

- Grains, including flours made from grains (wheat, rice, barley, millet, rye, spelt, corn, popcorn)—except occasional steel-cut oatmeal for breakfast

- Pasta, bread, crackers, cookies, flour, and cereal

- French fries

- Fruit juice

- Pineapple, banana, grapes, raisins, and bottled or canned fruit or fruit juice

- Fast food and soft drinks

- Sweetened yogurt and kefir, whole and 2 percent milk and ice cream

- Glucose, dextrose, sucrose, corn syrup, honey, sugar, maple syrup, or maltodextrin

- Diet drinks and artificial sweeteners

- Hydrogenated vegetable oil, margarine, Crisco, commercial mayo, and salad dressing

- MSG (monosodium glutamate) in soups or any other foods

- Canola oil

- Peanuts and peanut food products

Treats and cheats (for weekends only; best to eat before 3:00 p.m.; commit to this program for thirty days before cheating)

- ½ cup of whole fruit (allowable fruits are grapefruit, whole oranges, kiwi, strawberries, cranberries, watermelon, raspberries, peaches, blueberries, blackberries, and apricots)

- ½ cup of certain whole grains (allowable whole grains are brown rice pasta, fiber crisp crackers, 100 percent buckwheat Japanese soba noodles, and organic brown rice)

- Potato (allowable potatoes are half of a baked potato with one pat of organic butter, half of a serving of mashed potatoes, and homemade french fries made from stir-frying potato wedges in coconut butter)

- Refried beans made with extra-virgin olive oil

SIMPLE RULES

The following are simple dieting rules that I always recommend to my patients who need to lose weight, especially belly fat:

1. Graze throughout the day. (Eat lots of salads and veggies often throughout the day.)

2. Eat a large breakfast. Eat breakfast like a king, lunch like a prince, and dinner like a pauper.

3. Eat smaller midmorning and midafternoon snacks, such as recommended protein bars and coconut milk kefir blended with Life's Basics Plant Protein.

4. Avoid all simple sugar foods such as candies, cookies, cakes, pies, and doughnuts. If you must have sugar, use either stevia, Sweet Balance, or Just Like Sugar (found in health food stores.)

5. Drink two quarts of filtered or bottled water a day. It is best to drink two 8-oz. glasses thirty minutes before each meal, or one to two 8-oz. glasses two and a half hours after each meal, and 8 to 16 oz. upon waking.

6. Avoid alcohol.

7. Avoid all fried foods.

8. Avoid, or decrease dramatically, starches. Starches include all breads, crackers, bagels, potatoes, pasta, rice, and corn. Limit beans to ½ cup one to two times a day. Also avoid bananas and dried fruit.

9. Eat fresh low-glycemic fruits only for breakfast or lunch; steamed, stir-fried, or raw vegetables; lean meats; salads (preferably with extra-virgin olive oil and vinegar); almonds and seeds.

10. Take fiber supplements such as one to three capsules of PGX fiber with 16 oz. of water before each meal. (See appendix.)

11. For snacks, choose bars such as Jay Robb bars, gluten-free bars, and chocolate flaxseed bars. Try to limit these bars to one or two a day. These

may be purchased at a health food store. Refer to *Dr. Colbert's "I Can Do This" Diet* for more information.

12. Do not eat past 7:00 p.m.

> For God has not given us a spirit of fear and timidity, but of power, love, and self-discipline.
> —2 TIMOTHY 1:7

I strongly recommend my book *Dr. Colbert's "I Can Do This" Diet* for weight loss. Start every day with prayer to God for success. Speak aloud the Bible verses that are scattered throughout this book. In addition, plan your menu each day, and follow these additional simple rules. With a little patience, you'll be well on your way to that slimmer person you pictured when you closed your eyes—the healthy person God intended you to be!

FAITH MOVES MOUNTAINS

Feel like you've got a mountain of extra weight to lose? Don't be discouraged. You did not gain it overnight, and losing it overnight would not be healthy. Jesus Christ taught that any mountain of bondage will move when faith is applied. Look at the verse: "'You don't have enough faith,' Jesus told them. 'I tell you the truth, if you had faith even as small as a mustard seed, you could say to this mountain, "Move from here to there," and it would move. Nothing would be impossible'" (Matt. 17:20).

Let me teach you something about faith. Faith is the most

powerful force in the universe. Absolutely nothing is impossible to a person with faith. Faith is a belief that you already have what you are believing for. "[He] calls those things which do not exist as though they did" (Rom. 4:17, NKJV). Your daily vision and your daily confession then feed your faith. Your faith is similar to planting a seed, and the vision and confession are the seeds receiving nutrients—sunshine and water. On the other hand, getting discouraged and speaking defeat is similar to digging up your seed. Listen carefully: Faith is not a feeling or an emotion. It is a choice—a decision to believe God's Word despite everything else to the contrary. I have watched faith move many mountains. I have seen many people rise from wheelchairs and be healed by the power of the Holy Spirit. They were no different from you. They didn't think higher thoughts or come from more godly families. However, they did choose to believe God, to have a vision of themselves healed, and to make a daily confession of their healing. It's so simple.

Choose faith, and apply it right now to your situation.

A **BIBLE CURE** Prayer for You

Lord, I surrender the entire issue of weight control to You. Help me to face this issue in my life and find new hope, fresh vision, and powerful victory in You. Your Word says, "Nothing is impossible with God." I choose to believe Your Word right now and surrender and cast down all my feelings and thoughts of defeat in the arena of weight control. Thank You for loving me just as I am. And thank You for helping me to control my weight so that I will live a longer and better life. Amen.

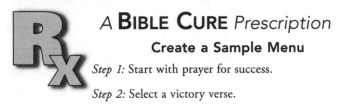

A **BIBLE CURE** *Prescription*

Create a Sample Menu

Step 1: Start with prayer for success.

Step 2: Select a victory verse.

Step 3: Today's menu based upon the allowable foods from my Rapid Waist Reduction Diet:

Breakfast:

_____

_____

_____

Lunch:

_____

_____

_____

Dinner:

_____

_____

_____

Snacks:

_____

_____

_____

In addition, I will implement the following simple rules:

- Graze throughout the day. (Eat lots of salads and veggies often throughout the day.)
- Eat a large breakfast.
- Eat smaller midmorning and midafternoon snacks.
- Avoid all simple sugar foods such as candies, cookies, cakes, pies, and doughnuts.
- Drink two quarts of filtered or bottled water a day.
- Other:

_____

_____

_____

_____

_____

_____

BATTLE DIABETES WITH NUTRIENTS AND SUPPLEMENTS

THERE ARE GOD-CREATED ways for you to add nutrients and supplements to your diet to begin controlling your blood sugar in a systematic, natural way. Both type 1 and type 2 diabetes can be helped by nutritional supplements. You must remember that supplements cannot take the place of a complete program to control and reverse type 2 diabetes that includes a focus on weight reduction, a good dietary plan, a regular exercise program, as well as stress reduction and hormone replacement therapy.

Following is a complete list of nutrients and supplements that will help you fight type 2 diabetes. (If you have type 1 diabetes, these supplements are still helpful to your overall health; however, the supplements listed below that will be of greatest benefit in fighting your form of diabetes are alpha lipoic acid, vitamin D, chromium, PGX fiber, omega 3, and the supplements for decreasing glycation.)

A good multivitamin

The foundation of a good supplement program always starts with a good comprehensive multivitamin. Adequate doses of nutrients found in a good multivitamin include magnesium, vanadium, biotin and the B vitamins, and the macro minerals and trace minerals.

- Magnesium is essential for glucose balance and is important for the release of insulin and the maintenance of the pancreatic beta cells, which produce insulin. Magnesium also increases the affinity and number of insulin receptors, which are on the surface of cells. The recommended daily allowance for magnesium is 350 mg a day for men and 280 mg a day for women.

- Vanadium is another mineral that assists in the metabolism of glucose.

- Biotin is a B vitamin that helps prevent insulin resistance.

Even though a multivitamin is extremely important in forming the foundation of a nutritional supplement program, there are other key nutrients or a larger dose of certain vitamins and minerals that you need to take in addition to a good comprehensive multivitamin. Most physicians are unaware of which nutritional supplements are effective in lowering blood sugar levels. You will need to make your physician aware that you are taking supplements for diabetes. The supplements alone are able to lower one's blood sugar significantly, and diabetic medication dosages will eventually need to be lowered accordingly. However, when the nutritional supplements are combinded with weight loss, regular exercise, my dietary program, stress reduction, and hormone replacement, the results are typically profound.

Vitamin D

Many Americans are not getting enough vitamin D, and we are beginning to see a close link between vitamin D deficiency and diabetes. A recent article published by researchers from Loyola University's Marcella Niehoff School of Nursing concluded that an adequate intake of vitamin D may prevent or delay the onset of diabetes as well as decrease complications for those who are diagnosed with diabetes. This article substantiated the role of vitamin D in the prevention as well as management of glucose intolerance and diabetes.[1]

Vitamin D also plays an important role in the secretion of insulin and in helping you avoid insulin resistance. Vitamin D not only decreases your blood sugar but also increases your body's sensitivity to insulin, thus make insulin more effective.

I check vitamin D levels on most of my patients by checking the 25-OHD3 level. I typically try to get the patient's vitamin D level greater than fifty and less than one hundred. I typically start most of my patients on 2,000 IU of vitamin D a day and may increase that amount to 4,000 or even 6,000 IU a day as I continue to monitor their 25-OHD3 level until the vitamin D level is greater than fifty. I then place them on a maintenance dose of vitamin D.

Chromium

Chromium is a mineral that is essential for good health. It has been of interest to diabetes researchers for a long time because it is required for normal metabolism of sugar, carbs, protein, and fat. Chromium is like insulin's little helper, and without adequate chromium, insulin cannot function properly.

How much chromium do you need? In 1989, the National

Academy of Sciences recommended an intake range for adults and adolescents of 50 to 200 mcg of chromium daily.[2] The Food and Nutrition Board of the Institute of Medicine has since narrowed this range down to 35 mcg for men and 25 mcg for women ages nineteen to fifty.[3]

A well-balanced diet should always be your first step in getting adequate amounts of vitamins, minerals, and other nutrients; however, fewer and fewer foods are providing the needed dietary intake levels of this important mineral. Whole grains and mushrooms may contain trace amounts of chromium, but that is only if these foods are grown in soils containing chromium. Likewise, seafood and some meat contain chromium, but only if the foods the animals ate contained chromium. Brewer's yeast is the only natural food source high in chromium; however, very few people eat this on a regular basis.

Also the standard American diet, full of refined sugars and carbohydrates, actually *depletes* your body of chromium since these foods require chromium for metabolism. I recommend you avoid foods high in refined sugars and carbs and consider taking chromium in supplement form.

Type 2 diabetics in particular tend to be deficient in chromium, whether as a cause or result of their condition. For this reason, I especially recommend supplementing chromium if you have type 2 diabetes.

A **BIBLE CURE** *Health Fact*

Selected Food Sources of Chromium[4]

A well-balanced diet does provide you with some chromium; however, the methods used for growing and manufacturing certain foods greatly affect their chromium levels and make it difficult to determine specific amounts of chromium you receive from each food. The following chart shows approximate chromium levels in foods, but it should only be used as a general guide.

Food	Chromium (mcg)
Broccoli, ½ cup	11
Grape juice, 1 cup	8
English muffin, whole wheat, 1	4
Potatoes, mashed, 1 cup	3
Garlic, dried, 1 teaspoon	3
Basil, dried, 1 tablespoon	2
Beef cubes, 3 ounces	2
Orange juice, 1 cup	2
Turkey breast, 3 ounces	2
Whole wheat bread, 2 slices	2
Red wine, 5 ounces	1–13
Apple, unpeeled, 1 medium	1
Banana, 1 medium	1
Green beans, ½ cup	1

Richard A. Anderson, PhD, chief chemist at the USDA Nutrient Requirements and Functions Laboratory, has conducted many studies on chromium supplementation and its effects on diabetes. He says, "Increased intake of chromium has been shown to lead to improvements in glucose, insulin, lipids, and related variables."[5]

Be aware that chromium is commonly included in multivitamins, usually in amounts ranging from 100 to 200 mcg. For many people this may provide adequate supplementation.[6] Always inform your doctor before making any changes to your diet or supplement program; however, realize that most doctors are unaware of this information.

There are several forms of chromium used for supplementation, but the most common form is chromium picolinate. For my type 2 diabetic patients, I typically recommend supplementing chromium picolinate in the amount of 600 to 1,000 mcg a day in divided doses.

One study conducted by Dr. Anderson found that type 2 diabetics who consumed 1,000 mcg per day of chromium improved insulin sensitivity without significant changes in body fat; type 1 diabetics were able to reduce their insulin dosage by 30 percent after only ten days of supplemental chromium picolinate at 200 mcg per day.[7]

Other studies in which researchers gave chromium to people with type 1 and type 2 diabetes have yielded mixed results. However, Dr. Anderson says that studies that show no beneficial effects using chromium for diabetes were usually using doses of chromium of 200 mcg or less, which is simply inadequate for diabetes, especially if the chromium is in the form that is poorly absorbed.[8]

Can you take too much chromium? According to Dr. Anderson's research, no discernible toxicity has been found in rats that consumed levels up to several thousand times the dietary reference for chromium for humans (based on body weight). There have also been no documented toxic effects in any of the human studies involving supplemental chromium, according to Dr. Anderson.[9] But again, please don't take massive amounts of any supplement without the advice of your doctor.

Alpha lipoic acid

Alpha lipoic acid is an important nutrient for fighting both type 1 and type 2 diabetes. Diabetics are more prone to oxidative stress and free radical formation than nondiabetics. Lipoic acid is an amazing antioxidant that works in both water-soluble and fat-soluble compartments of the body and regenerates vitamin C, vitamin E, coenzyme Q_{10}, and glutathione. Lipoic acid also improves insulin resistance in overweight adults suffering from type 2 diabetes.

Lipoic acid can also help relieve several components of metabolic syndrome: it can lower blood pressure, decrease insulin resistance, improve the lipid profile, and help individuals lose weight. Lipoic acid has also been used in Europe for decades to treat diabetic neuropathy with amazing success.

I usually start my diabetic patients on 300 mg of alpha lipoic acid twice a day, monitoring their blood sugars, and I may occasionally go up to 300 mg three times a day. Some patients develop GI side effects, skin allergies, or decreased thyroid function, so I monitor these tests closely while a patient is taking lipoic acid. Scientific studies using doses ranging from 300 mg to 1,800 mg a day infer that the most important form of lipoic acid is R-dihydro-lipoic acid, which is the most readily available form.[10] However, I find that alpha lipoic acid usually works best for the diabetic patients I have treated.

Cinnamon

The Chinese have used cinnamon medicinally for over four thousand years. Ancient Egyptians and Romans also recognized its many uses, and it has remained one of the most common spices in the world to this day.

In recent years, cinnamon's therapeutic effects have made headlines as some research has shown that cinnamon may have an insulin-like effect and cause blood sugar to be stored in the form of glycogen. It also contains excellent antioxidant properties.

The most commonly cited study on the effects of cinnamon in diabetes was published in *Diabetes Care* in 2003. Sixty people with type 2 diabetes were divided into six groups of ten patients each. Groups one through three were treated with 1, 3, or 6 g of cinnamon per day, and groups four through six received a placebo. After forty days, the cinnamon group's reduction in blood sugar was amazing. Their fasting blood sugars were lowered by 18 to 29 percent. The placebo group, however, showed no change.[11]

Whole cinnamon contains oils that may trigger allergic reactions. This is why I recommend a cinnamon extract instead. One form of cinnamon extract is Cinnulin PF, which contains the active component found in whole cinnamon without the toxins. USDA studies have indicated that cinnamon extract promotes glucose metabolism and healthy cholesterol levels in people with type 2 diabetes.[12] Cinnamon extract also appears to help glucose transport mechanisms by increasing the insulin signaling pathways. I generally recommend taking 250 mg of Cinnulin PF twice a day.

Soluble fiber

As I mentioned in chapter 2, soluble fiber not only helps to slow the digestion of starches, but it also slows glucose uptake and thus lowers the glycemic index of your meal. This in turn lowers the amount of insulin that is secreted by the pancreas, which is very beneficial for those with type 2 diabetes. Soluble fiber has also been shown over the years through numerous studies to effectively lower blood sugar levels.[13]

How does it do all of these things? Soluble fiber actually swells many times its original size as it binds to the water in your stomach and small intestine to form a gluelike gel that not only slows down the absorption of glucose but also induces a sense of satiety (fullness) and reduces your body's absorption of calories.

High-fiber diets

Studies conducted by James W. Anderson, MD, of the University of Kentucky, showed that high-fiber diets lowered insulin requirements an average of 38 percent in people with type 1 diabetes and 97 percent in people with type 2 diabetes. This means that almost all of the people suffering from type 2 diabetes who followed Dr. Anderson's high-fiber diet were able to lower or stop taking insulin and other diabetes medications and still maintain a healthy blood sugar level. Additionally, these results lasted up to fifteen years.[14]

Fruit, beans, chickpeas, lentils, carrots, squash, oat bran, barley, rice bran, guar gum, glucomannan, and pectin are all very good sources of soluble fiber.

Supplementing with PGX

Of course, in addition to dietary sources of fiber, it's a good idea to supplement. I recommend a specific fiber supplement developed by scientists at the University of Toronto called PGX (short for PolyGlycopleX). Often called the new "super fiber," PGX is a unique blend of plant fibers containing glucomannan, a soluble and fermentable fiber derived from the root of the konjac plant. It also contains sodium alginate, xanthan gum, and mulberry leaf extract. It works the same as dietary sources of fiber; however, the specific ratio of natural compounds used in PGX enable it to be three to five times as effective as other fibers alone.

Clinical studies by Dr. Vuksan, the developer of PGX, have shown repeatedly that blood sugar levels after meals decrease as soluble fiber viscosity increases.[15] The exciting news is that PGX fiber lowers after-meal blood sugars by approximately 20 percent and also lowers insulin secretion by approximately 40 percent. This is unequaled by any drug or natural health-food product.

Recently, researchers at the University of Toronto found that higher doses of PGX can decrease appetite significantly because PGX absorbs six hundred times its weight in water over one to two hours and expands in the digestive tract.[16]

Most soluble fiber has side effects of producing significant amounts of gas; however, PGX has fewer GI side effects than other dietary fiber, mainly because PGX can be given in much smaller quantities than other viscous fibers and achieve comparable health benefits without all the gas.[17]

Any time you increase your fiber intake, you should start slowly and drink plenty of water. With PGX, I recommend that you start with one capsule, three times a day before meals, with 16 oz. of water, and gradually increase the dose as tolerated every two to three days. Most people use two to three softgels before meals with 16 oz. of water. Rarely will someone need six softgels before meals, which is the maximum dose.

Irvingia

Irvingia is a fruit-bearing plant from the jungles of Cameroon. It is believed that Irvingia has the ability to enable one to lose weight by simply lowering CRP (C-reactive protein) levels, which in turn lowers leptin resistance.[18]

Leptin is a hormone that tells your brain you've eaten enough and it's time to stop. It also enhances your body's ability to use fat as an energy source.

Unfortunately, because of sedentary lifestyles and the many highly processed, high-glycemic food choices available through the standard American diet, many overweight and obese patients have acquired resistance to leptin, and this hormone no longer works properly in their bodies. Similar to insulin resistance, leptin resistance is a chronic inflammatory condition that contributes to weight gain as well as belly fat.

This is why the new research demonstrating Irvingia's promise in reversing leptin resistance is so important. In one double-blind study, 102 overweight volunteers took either 150 mg of Irvingia or a placebo twice a day for ten weeks. At the end of ten weeks, the Irvingia group lost on average of 28 pounds with 6.7 inches lost from their waistlines. The Irvingia group also had a 32 percent reduction in fasting blood sugar, 26 percent reduction in total cholesterol, and 52 percent reduction in CRP.[19]

I have been using Irvingia with my diabetic patients since 2008 and have seen remarkable improvements in most of their blood sugar measurements as well their hemoglobin A1C levels. The dose that is generally recommended is 150 mg of standardized Irvingia extract two times a day.

Omega-3 fatty acids

Omega-3 fats are simply polyunsaturated fats that come from foods such as fish, fish oil, vegetable oils (especially flaxseed oil), walnuts, and wheat germ. However, the most beneficial omega-3 fats are fish oils containing EPA and DHA.

Omega-3 fats generally protect against heart disease, decrease inflammation, lower triglyceride levels, and may help prevent insulin resistance and improve glucose tolerance. Fish oil also helps to decrease the rate of developing diabetic vascular complications. Omega-3 fats also decrease inflammation, help to reduce the risk of heart disease and stroke, and slow the progression of atherosclerosis.

Even though fish oils are probably the most protective fats for our blood vessels, trans fats are actually the worst fats for our blood vessels and also can greatly increase one's risk of developing diabetes. Trans fats are hydrogenated fats or partially hydrogenated fats and are ubiquitous in both processed and fast food as well as served in many restaurants and restaurant chains. A recent study showed that only a 2 percent increase in calories from trans fat raised the risk of diabetes in females by 39 percent, and a 5 percent increase in polyunsaturated fats decreased the risk of diabetes by 37 percent.[20]

Dietary fats that are considered to be beneficial include not only fish oils but also avocados, extra-virgin olive oil, almond butter, nuts, and seeds.

A word of caution since some fish oil supplements may

contain mercury, pesticides, or PCBs. See the appendix for fish oil (omega-3) products I recommend as safe.

I usually place my patients with prediabetes and those with diabetes on 320 to 1,000 mg of fish oils three times a day. If they have high triglyceride levels, I may increase the dose to 4,000 to 5,000 mg a day.

SUPPLEMENTS TO DECREASE GLYCATION

Carnosine

Glycation is the name for protein molecules that bind to glucose molecules and form advanced glycation end products (AGEs). Glycated proteins produce fifty times more free radicals than nonglycated proteins. Typical manifestations of this are skin wrinkling and brain degeneration. Both prediabetics and diabetics are much more prone to glycation and, as a result, will age prematurely.

The amino acid carnosine, however, helps stabilize and protect cell membranes from glycation. Carnosine is a safe and effective nutrient for inhibiting glycation. I usually recommend at least 1,000 mg a day of carnosine to my diabetic patients.

Pyridoxamine

A unique form of vitamin B_6 called pyridoxamine interferes with accelerated glycation reactions in diabetics. Glycation end products are closely linked with diabetic kidney disease, diabetic retinopathy, and diabetic neuropathy. However, pyridoxamine is one of the most powerful natural supplements for inhibiting AGE formation and has been found to be superior to the other two forms of vitamin B_6 in inhibiting AGE formation and glycation.

> Do not carouse with drunkards or feast with gluttons, for they are on their way to poverty, and too much sleep clothes them in rags.
> —PROVERBS 23:20–21

Pyridoxamine has been studied clinically in the treatment of diabetic kidney disease. Trials at the Joslin Diabetes Center at Harvard Medical School are promising using pyridoxamine and suggest a protective effect of kidney function in diabetics.[21]

Neurological problems can occur when you consume megadoses (more than 2,000 mg per day); therefore, I recommend you stay on the safe side with a dose of 50 mg (one capsule) of pyridoxamine, taken with food once a day.

Benfotiamine

Benfotiamine is a fat-soluble form of vitamin B_1 and has been shown to help prevent the development as well as progression of many diabetic complications. This has been used in Europe for decades as a prescription medication. It helps to slow the progression of diabetic nerve, kidney, and retinal disease, and also helps to relieve diabetic neuropathy. Benfotiamine is fat soluble, so it can easily enter cells and help prevent dysfunction associated with diabetes within the cells.

A recent double-blind study in Germany found that diabetic patients with polyneuropathy who were given 100 mg of benfotiamine four times a day for three weeks had statistically significant improvement in nerve function scores.[22]

Benfotiamine offers protection for the nerves, kidneys, retina, and vascular system from damage caused by diabetes. That is why supplementation is extremely important in preventing long-term complications of type 1 and type 2 diabetes. My recommended dose is 100 mg four times a day.

A BIBLE CURE *Health Tip*
Dr. Colbert's Diabetic Protocol

I place all of my diabetic patients on a comprehensive multivitamin, as well as omega-3 fat. I also typically place them on vitamin D, chromium, alpha lipoic acid, cinnulin, Irvingia, and PGX fiber. I generally will add a supplement to prevent glycation such as carnosine, pyridoxamine, or benfotiamine. I usually start pyridoxamine if they are developing symptoms of glycation, such as kidney disease, neuropathy, or retinopathy. For more information on supplements as well as more in-depth dietary and exercise information, please refer to my book *The Seven Pillars of Health*.

SUPPLEMENTS TO REPLENISH HORMONES

Balancing hormones is extremely important in managing diabetes. Elevated stress hormone levels are associated with increased belly fat and increased insulin resistance, causing decreased blood sugar control. Sex hormone deficiency has actually decreased the effectiveness of insulin. It is interesting to note that aging is associated with a decrease in sex hormone levels and an increase in the incidence of type 2 diabetes.

Testosterone

Testosterone is the male hormone that is associated with increased muscle mass, deepening of the voice, and male pattern hair growth. High testosterone levels are associated with a significantly lower risk of type 2 diabetes in men. On the other hand, low levels of testosterone in males have repeatedly been shown to be associated with an increased risk of type 2 diabetes as well as abdominal obesity.

> Let all that I am praise the LORD; with my whole heart, I will praise his holy name. Let all that I am praise the LORD; may I never forget the good things he does for me. He forgives all my sins and heals all my diseases.
>
> —Psalm 103:1–3

Testosterone replacement therapy decreases insulin resistance and improves blood sugar control in men with low testosterone levels. In all men with type 2 diabetes, I always check both total and free testosterone levels, and I have found that a large percentage of men with type 2 diabetes indeed have low testosterone levels. I then typically place them on a small amount of transdermal testosterone cream in order to raise their testosterone levels to normal. To find a doctor knowledgeable in hormone replacement therapy (HRT), please see the appendix.

It is interesting to note that high testosterone levels are also associated with a higher risk of type 2 diabetes in females. I believe the reason for this is that many women with high testosterone levels also have large waist measurements or increased belly fat.

Also, women with high testosterone levels may have polycystic ovary syndrome (PCOS). PCOS runs in families and is associated with insulin resistance; infertility; increased hair on the face, arms, and legs; acne; obesity; and elevated testosterone levels. They are also at a significant increased risk of developing type 2 diabetes.

PCOS gets its name from early cases that were associated with multiple cysts of the ovaries. However, this is not a main feature of this condition even though the name has stuck.

It is also interesting to note that PCOS can be managed with a very low glycemic diet as well as exercise. Many physicians also use the diabetic medication metformin, which helps control the blood sugar.

A BIBLE CURE *Health Tip*

Medications for Polycystic Ovary Syndrome[23]

Because there is no cure for PCOS, it needs to be managed very carefully. Most physicians prescribe a combination of treatments based on their specific symptoms. These treatments include birth control pills, diabetes medications, antiandrogens to decrease the impact of male hormones, and even surgery.

Research shows that more than 50 percent of women with PCOS are likely to have prediabetes or diabetes before the age of forty. Keeping the symptoms of PCOS under control is the best way to reduce your risk of developing complications like diabetes, heart disease, and cancer. Regular testing for diabetes, eating right, exercising, and not smoking are also very helpful in reducing your chances of developing serious health problems associated with PCOS. Also, the supplements for type 2 diabetes will also help PCOS, but diet and regular exercise are absolutely critical for managing it.

Estrogen

It is interesting to note that when many women go through menopause, they typically develop a *menopot*, or potbelly, as well as increased truncal obesity. As their weight gradually increases, their cholesterol typically increases, their blood pressure usually rises, and their blood sugar level also typically rises.

If you are a woman, a very important function of estrogen is that it fights insulin resistance by improving the effectiveness of insulin, helping to lower your blood sugar. Estrogen also helps redistribute the fat from your waist to your hips, buttocks, and thigh areas. Estrogen increases your metabolic rate and helps you maintain muscle mass as well.

In other words, estrogen helps prevent diabetes. But unfortunately, most doctors do not prescribe transdermal bioidentical estrogen but synthetic estrogen in pill form, such as Premarin (a prescription estrogen medication made from pregnant mare's urine), which causes more weight gain and a greater risk of diabetes. Premarin is the most common prescribed estrogen and is associated with weight gain. I've helped so many women over the years control their blood sugar and lose weight by balancing their hormones with bioidentical transdermal hormone creams. To find a doctor knowledgeable in HRT in your area, please refer to the appendix.

Progesterone

In women, it is also critically important to balance estrogen with progesterone, the other female hormone. Progesterone actually helps to balance estrogen levels. Progesterone also has a natural calming effect on the body and helps one to sleep. This helps to lower cortisol levels, which will also help lower blood sugar levels.

However, most women are taking synthetic progesterone, such as Provera, or taking large doses of bioidentical progesterone. When women take either synthetic progesterone or too much natural progesterone, it decreases glucose tolerance or may predispose one to developing diabetes. Progesterone can also increase insulin and cortisol levels, setting you up for increased belly fat and rising blood sugar levels.

Now, hopefully you are beginning to understand the importance of balancing these very important hormones and checking the levels of these hormones.

> Wise words satisfy like a good meal; the right words bring satisfaction. The tongue can bring death or life; those who love to talk will reap the consequences.
> —PROVERBS 18:20–21

A FINAL NOTE

As you have observed, there are many nutrients and supplements that can help you effectively battle diabetes. If you are a type 2 diabetic and you choose to follow this program and monitor your blood sugar, you should find that your blood sugar is likely to drop within the normal range in a few months.

If you are a type 1 diabetic, until you receive complete divine healing from God, you will always be on insulin. However, you may be able to lower your dosage of insulin by following the measures outlined in this book.

Regularly consult with your physician, and use these vitamins and nutrients as he or she may recommend. God has created these wonderful natural substances to empower us in maintaining good health and overcoming the debilitating effects of diabetes.

A **BIBLE CURE** Prayer for You

Heavenly Father, help me apply these things I have learned in my battle against diabetes. Help me eat wisely and obtain my ideal body weight. Show me which vitamins, minerals, and supplements will best help my body fight diabetes. Heal my body so that insulin will be produced and then used by my cells in a healthy way. Strengthen my resolve to exercise regularly. Keep me in Your divine health so that I may live a long, productive life serving You. Amen.

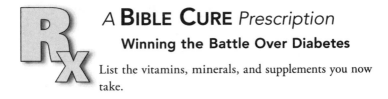

A **BIBLE CURE** Prescription
Winning the Battle Over Diabetes

List the vitamins, minerals, and supplements you now take.

_____

_____

_____

_____

What supplements do you plan to add in order to treat diabetes?

_____

_____

_____

_____

If you are a male, have you had your total and free testosterone levels checked? If you are a female and are menopausal or premenopausal, have you had your hormone levels checked? Are you taking synthetic estrogen or synthetic progesterone in pill form? If so, see a doctor knowledgeable in bioidentical hormones.

_____

_____

_____

_____

BATTLE DIABETES WITH SPIRITUAL AND EMOTIONAL STRENGTH

HAVE YOU BEEN told that you have diabetes? As a Christian physician, I can tell you that you do need to believe God for a miracle. Balanced with that, it is necessary for you to do your part to take care of your health. But if miracles happened every time we wanted them to happen, they wouldn't be miracles anymore—they would be cures!

Miracles are a divine touch, a moment of supernatural intervention when total healing occurs—but all healing is from God. A doctor can sew up an incision and bind up a wound. But the power that heals the wound and makes you well again always comes from God. I encourage you to pray for a miracle, but don't stop there. Lay hold of the principles of health outlined in this book to aid the healing process. In addition, let's look at diabetes in another way that you may not have thought of.

ANOTHER DIMENSION

Throughout this book we have taken a close look at the physical side of diabetes. But another dimension exists to this disease that we must also address: a spiritual and emotional dimension.

> A merry heart does good, like medicine, but a broken
> spirit dries the bones.
>
> —PROVERBS 17:22, NKJV

The Bible strongly suggests that our health sometimes has an emotional and spiritual component. Do you know that negative emotions can affect your physical body? According to the Bible, they can.

LESS STRESS

One significant factor that will elevate your insulin level and make you vulnerable to diabetes is stress. As I discuss in my book *Stress Less*, it is common for people under chronic stress to have elevated leves of cortisol and insulin. At normal levels, cortisol (your body's stress hormone) counterbalances the effects of insulin. However, elevated cortisol decreases your sensitivity to insulin, which leads to insulin resistance.

In addition, elevated cortisol levels stimulate your appetite, producing a craving for sugars and carbohydrates—the very foods that keep your insulin levels elevated. By creating this vicious cycle, you can see how living with chronic stress programs your body for fat storage and obesity, and unfortunately, metabolic syndrome, prediabetes, and type 2 diabetes often follow.

God's plan is for you to handle stress by casting your cares on Him. "Give all your worries and cares to God, for he cares about you" (1 Pet. 5:7).

What cares have you neglected to give to God?

- Financial concerns
- Hurting relationships
- Future goals
- Job-related anxieties
- Other: _____

God cares for you and wants to see you through all the stress and worry you may be facing. If you hold on to your stress, then your body will suffer. Surrender your cares to Him.

TAKE THESE BIBLE CURE STEPS

I discuss the following stress busters in greater detail in my books *Stress Less* and *The Seven Pillars of Health.* But as I close this Bible Cure book, I'd like to briefly suggest the following steps to eliminate as much stress as possible from your life and greatly reduce the risks and complications of diabetes.

Enjoy the present moment.

This concept, often called "mindfulness," is the practice of learning to pay attention to what is happening to you from moment to moment. The definition of mindfulness reminds me of the words of Jesus:

> Therefore do not worry about tomorrow, for tomorrow will worry about its own things. Sufficient for the day is its own trouble.
>
> —MATTHEW 6:34, NKJV

Replace stress and worry about the future (or the past) with something to enjoy in the present moment.

Reframe your thinking.

While mindfulness is learning to live in the present moment, reframing is learning to see the past, present, and future in a positive light. When negative beliefs or thoughts pop up, challenge and assess them rather than automatically accepting them. This is what the apostle Paul meant when he said:

> Casting down imaginations, and every high thing that exalteth itself against the knowledge of God, and bringing into captivity every thought to the obedience of Christ.
> —2 CORINTHIANS 10:5, KJV, EMPHASIS ADDED

This is simply replacing your fears, worries, failures, grief, sorrows, and shame with God's promises. Reframing your thoughts in this way will lower your stress level and have a very real effect on your body.

Build margin into your life.

A very practical way to de-stress your life is to build margin into everything you do. Margin is a buffer between feeling overwhelmed and feeling at peace. Allowing yourself two hours to get to the airport when you only need one hour is margin. When you make a budget and only spend 80 percent of what you earn, that's margin.

Margin will not automatically appear in your schedule or finances. You must plan it and put it there. Learn to cut back on commitments, manage your time better, make a to-do list every night for the following day, build in time between appointments, spend less than you earn, pay off credit cards, and build up an emergency fund. These things will all build margin into your life, and your stress level will go down dramatically.

Remove obvious stressors, and surround yourself with positive people.

If you are under stress, it's likely that your environment includes stressors that can be removed. These might include clutter, an overcrowded schedule, or your relationships. Restoring order to your home or work environment is a proven stress reducer and slams the door on stress.

Now, I realize you can't completely avoid negative people or relationships, but I strongly encourage you to limit the amount of time you spend with them. Attitudes are contagious. Don't let their negative attitude drain all of your energy, joy, and strength. Instead, surround yourself with positive friends whose attitudes and words are those of love, thankfulness, appreciation, and humility.

Learn the power of "no."

Learning to say no is hard for some people, but it is very important. When you protect your time and energy because you realize how infinitely valuable they are to your mind, body, and spirit, you will avoid the stress that comes from overcommitting yourself and taking on problems or goals that are not your own. Instead, learn to assertively stand behind your own visions and goals for your life. Create healthy boundaries, and enforce them. You will find that your confidence increases as you do this, and your stress level will drop.

Pray.

Prayer is an unlimited resource for filling your life with God's Spirit, wisdom, strength, and peace. Philippians 4:6–7 says, "Be anxious for nothing, but in everything by prayer and supplication with thanksgiving let your requests be made known to God. And the peace of God, which surpasses all comprehension, will guard your hearts and your minds in Christ Jesus."

Meditate on God's Word.

Throughout this book are scriptures that will strengthen and encourage you. Learn them. Speak them aloud. Let His Word bring guidance and healing into your life.

> But his delight is in the law of the LORD, and in His law he meditates day and night. He shall be like a tree planted by the rivers of water, that brings forth its fruit in its season, whose leaf also shall not wither; and whatever he does shall prosper.
> —PSALM 1:2–3, NKJV

A **BIBLE CURE** Prayer for You

Heavenly Father, help me to apply all of these things I have learned. I take Your hand for the rest of my journey through the seasons of my life. Help me to walk in divine health throughout the path You lay before me and to know You better all along the way. Lord, help me to speak and think positive words so that my life will bring help and refreshing to others. Give me the power to stop destructive habits and attitudes. Fill me with Your joy for life, and give me energy to take the necessary steps to stay fit, both physically and spiritually all of my days. Amen.

A **BIBLE CURE** *Prescription*

What cares have you neglected to give to God, resulting in stress in your life?

❏ Financial concerns
❏ Hurting relationships
❏ Future goals
❏ Job-related anxieties
❏ Other: _____

Check the spiritual steps you have started in overcoming diabetes:

❏ I am enjoying the present moment.
❏ I am reframing my thoughts.
❏ I am building margin into my life.
❏ I am eliminating obvious stressors.
❏ I am surrounding myself with positive people.
❏ I am learning to say no.
❏ I am praying.
❏ I am learning and applying God's Word.
❏ I am trusting God for health and strength.

Write a prayer thanking God for all the ways He has created to help you overcome diabetes in your life:

_____

_____

_____

_____

_____

A PERSONAL NOTE
From Don Colbert

G OD DESIRES TO heal you of disease. His Word is full of promises that confirm His love for you and His desire to give you His abundant life. His desire includes more than physical health for you; He wants to make you whole in your mind and spirit as well as through a personal relationship with His Son, Jesus Christ.

If you haven't met my best friend, Jesus, I would like to take this opportunity to introduce Him to you. It is very simple. If you are ready to let Him come into your life and become your best friend, all you need to do is sincerely pray this prayer:

> *Lord Jesus, I want to know You as my Savior and Lord. I believe You are the Son of God and that You died for my sins. I also believe You were raised from the dead and now sit at the right hand of the Father praying for me. I ask You to forgive me for my sins and change my heart so that I can be Your child and live with You eternally. Thank You for Your peace. Help me to walk with You so that I can begin to know You as my best friend and my Lord. Amen.*

If you have prayed this prayer, you have just made the most important decision of your life. I rejoice with you in your decision and your new relationship with Jesus. Please contact my publisher at pray4me@charismamedia.com so that we can send you some materials that will help you become established in your relationship with the Lord. We look forward to hearing from you.

NUTRITIONAL SUPPLEMENTS FOR DIABETES

Divine Health Nutritional Products
1908 Boothe Circle
Longwood, FL 32750
Phone: (407) 331-7007
Web site: www.drcolbert.com
E-mail: info@drcolbert.com

Comprehensive multivitamin: Divine Health Multivitamin and Divine Health Living Multivitamin

Diabetic support: cinnulin, coffee berry, Divine Health Eye Sight, Divine Health Fiber, Divine Health Nutrients for Glucose Regulation, Irvingia, PGX fiber, pyridoxamine, Divine Health R Lipoic, Divine Health Vitamin D_3, and insulinase (cinnulin and chromium), benfotiamine, carnosine,

Omega Oils: Divine Health Omega Pure and Divine Health Living Omega

Metagenics
Alpha lipoic acid, 300 mg
(800) 692-9400 (refer to #W7741 when ordering)
www.drcolbert.meta-ehealth.com

WorldHealth.net
A global resource for antiaging medicine and to find a doctor that specializes in bioidentical hormone therapy

Life's Basics Protein

LifeTime Nutritional Specialties

www.lifetimevitamins.com/products/lifetime_plantprotein
.html

NOTES

INTRODUCTION

1. Diabetes Research Institute, "Diabetes Fact Sheet," http://www.diabetesresearch.org/Newsroom/DiabetesFactSheet (accessed July 28, 2009).

2. Centers for Disease Control and Prevention, "National Diabetes Fact Sheet," http://www.cdc.gov/diabetes/pubs/estimates.htm (accessed July 28, 2009).

3. World Health Organization, "What Is Diabetes?" http://www.who.int/mediacentre/factsheets/fs312/en/ (accessed July 28, 2009).

4. Centers for Disease Control and Prevention, "National Diabetes Fact Sheet."

5. Ibid.

6. Centers for Disease Control and Prevention, "Overweight Prevalence," http://www.cdc.gov/nchs/fastats/overwt.htm (accessed July 28, 2009).

CHAPTER 1
KNOW YOUR ENEMY

1. American Diabetes Association, "All About Diabetes," http://www.diabetes.org/about-diabetes.jsp (accessed July 28, 2009).

2. Ibid.

3. Centers for Disease Control and Prevention, "National Diabetes Fact Sheet."

4. American Diabetes Association, "A1C Test," http://www.diabetes.org/type-1-diabetes/a1c-test.jsp (accessed July 28, 2009).

5. Centers for Disease Control and Prevention, "National Diabetes Fact Sheet."

6. National Diabetes Information Clearinghouse, "National Diabetes Statistics, 2007," http://diabetes .niddk.nih.gov/dm/pubs/statistics/index .htm#complications (accessed July 28, 2009).

7. Centers for Disease Control and Prevention, "National Diabetes Fact Sheet."

8. The Diabetes Monitor, "Metabolic Syndrome," http:// www.diabetesmonitor.com/b429.htm (accessed July 29, 2009).

9. "Stress Treatments Helps Control Type 2 Diabetes," Mercola.com, http://articles.mercola.com/sites/articles/archive/2002/01/23/stress-treatments.aspx (accessed July 29, 2009).

10. Ibid.

11. National Diabetes Data Group and National Institutes of Health, *Diabetes in America*, 2nd edition (Bethesda, MD: National Institutes of Health, 1995).

12. National Institute of Neurological Diseases and Stroke, "Transient Ischemic Attack Information Page," http://www.ninds.nih.gov/disorders/tia/tia.htm (accessed July 29, 2009).

13. Centers for Disease Control and Prevention, "National Diabetes Fact Sheet."

14. National Eye Institute, "Diabetic Retinopathy," http://www.nei.nih.gov/health/diabetic/retinopathy.asp (accessed July 29, 2009).

15. Centers for Disease Control and Prevention, "National Diabetes Fact Sheet."

16. Ibid.

17. Ibid.

18. Ibid.

19. Ibid.

20. Ibid.

21. Ibid.

22. "Erectile Dysfunction (Impotence) and Diabetes," WebMD.com, http://www.webmd.com/erectile -dysfunction/guide/ed-diabetes (accessed July 29, 2009).

CHAPTER 2
BATTLE DIABETES WITH GOOD NUTRITION

1. National Institutes of Health Office of Dietary Supplements, "Dietary Supplement Fact Sheet: Calcium," http://ods.od.nih.gov/factsheets/Calcium_ pf.asp (accessed August 5, 2009).

2. Gabriel Cousens, *There Is a Cure for Diabetes* (Berkeley, CA: North Atlantic Books, 2008), 190–200.

3. Ibid., 179–182.

4. Dave Tuttle, "Controlling Blood Sugar With Cinnamon and Coffee Berry," *Life Extension* magazine, December 2005, as viewed online at http:// www.lef.org/magazine/mag2005/dec2005_report_ cinnamon_01.htm (accessed July 27, 2009).

5. Ibid.

6. Ibid.

CHAPTER 3
BATTLE DIABETES WITH ACTIVITY

1. Ming Wei, Larry W. Gibbons, Tedd L. Mitchell, James B. Kampert, Chong D. Lee, and Steven N. Blair, "The Association Between Cardiorespiratory Fitness and Impaired Fasting Glucose and Type 2 Diabetes Mellitus in Men," *Annals of Internal Medicine*, http://www.annals.org/cgi/content/abstract/130/2/89 (accessed July 29, 2009).

2. L. E. Davidson, R. Hudson, K. Kilpatrick, et al., "Effects of Exercise Modality on Insulin Resistance and Functional Limitation in Older Adults: a Randomized Controlled Trial," *Archives of Internal Medicine* 169, no. 2 (2009):122–131, as viewed online at http://archinte.ama-assn.org/cgi/content/abstract/169/2/122 on July 31, 2009.

CHAPTER 4
BATTLE DIABETES WITH WEIGHT LOSS

1. Centers for Disease Control and Prevention, "Defining Overweight and Obesity," http://www.cdc.gov/nccdphp/dnpa/obesity/defining.htm (accessed August 17, 2009).

2. Youfa Wang et al., "Comparison of Abdominal Adiposity and Overall Obesity in Predicting Risk of Type 2 Diabetes Among Men," *American Journal of Clinical Nutrition* 81, no. 3 (2005): 555–563.

CHAPTER 5
BATTLE DIABETES WITH NUTRIENTS AND SUPPLEMENTS

1. "Vitamin D Is the 'It' Nutrient of the Moment," ScienceDaily.com, http://www.sciencedaily.com/releases/2009/01/090112121821.htm (accessed July 30, 2009).

2. National Research Council, Food and Nutrition Board, *Recommended Dietary Allowances*, 10th edition (Washington DC: National Academy Press, 1989), as viewed online at http://ods.od.nih.gov/factsheets/chromium.asp#en17 (accessed July 27, 2009).

3. Neal D. Barnard, *Dr. Neal Barnard's Program for Reversing Diabetes* (New York: Rodale, 2007), 142.

4. National Institutes of Health Office of Dietary Supplements, "Dietary Supplement Fact Sheet: Chromium," http://ods.od.nih.gov/factsheets/chromium.asp (accessed July 27, 2009).

5. Richard Anderson, Noella Bryden, and Marilyn Polanski, "Chromium and Other Insuling Potentiators in the Prevention and Alleviation of Glucose Intolerance," United States Department of Agricultural Health, Agricultural Research Service, http://www.ars.usda.gov/research/publications/Publications.htm?seq_no_115=138818&pf=1 (accessed July 30, 2009).

6. Barnard, *Dr. Neal Barnard's Program for Reversing Diabetes*, 143.

7. Richard A. Anderson, "Chromium in the Prevention and Control of Diabetes," *Diabetes and Metabolism* (n.p., 2000), 22–27, as cited in Frank Murray, *Natural Supplements for Diabetes* (Laguna Beach, CA: Basic Health Publications, Inc. 2007), 114.

8. Ibid.

9. Richard A. Anderson, "Chromium, Glucose Intolerance and Diabetes" *Journal of the American College of Nutrition* 17, no. 6 (1998): 548–555, as viewed online at http://www.jacn.org/cgi/content/full/17/6/548 (accessed July 27, 2009).

10. Mark A. Mitchell, "Lipoic Acid: A Multitude of Metabolic Health Benefits," *Life Extension* magazine, October 2007, http://www.lef.org/LEFCMS/aspx/PrintVersionMagic.aspx?CmsID=115115 (accessed July 27, 2009).

11. John R. White, "Cinnamon: Should It Be Taken as a Diabetes Medication?" *Diabetes Health*, December 25, 2008. Accessed online at http://www.diabeteshealth.com/read/2008/12/25/5703/cinnamon-should-it-be-taken-as-a-diabetes-medication/ on July 27, 2009.

12. Mike Adams, "Study Shows Cinnulin Promotes Increase in Lean Body Mass and Reduction in Body Fat," NaturalNews.com, http://www.naturalnews.com/011852.html (accessed July 30, 2009).

13. Joslin Diabetes Center, "How Does Fiber Affect Blood Glucose Levels?" http://www.joslin.org/managing_your_diabetes_697.asp (accessed August 3, 2009).

14. James W. Anderson, *Dr. Anderson's High-Fiber Fitness Plan* (Lexington, KY: University Press of Kentucky, 1994), 14.

15. Michael Murray, "What Makes People Fat, Why Diets Don't Work, and What Triggers Appetite?" SmartBomb.com, http://www.smartbomb.com/drmurrayweight.html (accessed July 30, 2009).

16. "Good Bye to Fad Diets, Revolutionary Natural Fibre Discovered in Canada," MedicalNewsToday.com, http://www.medicalnewstoday.com/articles/12058.php (accessed July 30, 2009).

17. PGX, "Frequently Asked Questions," www.pgx.com/us/en/faq (accessed July 27, 2009).

18. Chris Lydon, "Turn Off Your Fat Switch: Understanding the Risks of Leptin Resistance," *Life Extension* magazine (April/May/June 2009), 49–55.

19. Ibid.

20. "Trans Fat, NOT Saturated Fat, Increases Diabetes," *American Journal of Nutrition* 73, (June 2001): 1001–1002, 1019–1026, as viewed at http://articles.mercola.com/sites/articles/archive/2001/06/16/diabetes-part-four.aspx (accessed August 3, 2009).

21. Laurie Barclay, "Unique Form of Vitamin B6 Protects Against Complications Related to Diabetes and Aging," *Life Extension* magazine, October 2008, as viewed online at http://www.lef.org/magazine/mag2008/oct2008_Vitamin-B6-Protects-Against-Diabetes-Aging_02.htm (accessed July 31, 2009).

22. Julius G. Goepp, "Protecting Against Glycation and High Blood Sugar With Benfotiamine," *Life Extension* magazine, April 2008, as viewed online at http://search.lef.org/cgi-src-bin/MsmGo .exe?grab_id=0&page_id=919&query=benfotiamine& hiword=BENFOTIAMIN%20BENFOTIAMINES% 20benfotiamine%20 (accessed July 31, 2009).

23. U. S. Department of Health and Human Services, "Polycystic Ovary Syndrome (PCOS)," WomensHealth.gov, http://www.womenshealth.gov/ faq/polycystic-ovary-syndrome.cfm (accessed July 31, 2009).

Don Colbert, MD, was born in Tupelo, Mississippi. He attended Oral Roberts School of Medicine in Tulsa, Oklahoma, where he received a bachelor of science degree in biology in addition to his degree in medicine. Dr. Colbert completed his internship and residency with Florida Hospital in Orlando, Florida. He is board certified in family practice and in anti-aging medicine and has received extensive training in nutritional medicine.

If you would like more information about natural and divine healing, or information about *Divine Health nutritional products*, you may contact Dr. Colbert at:

DON COLBERT, MD

1908 Boothe Circle
Longwood, FL 32750
Telephone: 407-331-7007 (for ordering product only)

Dr. Colbert's Web site is
www.drcolbert.com.

Disclaimer: Dr. Colbert and the staff of Divine Health Wellness Center are prohibited from addressing a patient's medical condition by phone, facsimile, or e-mail. Please refer questions related to your medical condition to your own primary care physician.

FREE NEWSLETTERS
TO HELP EMPOWER YOUR LIFE

Why subscribe today?

☐ **DELIVERED DIRECTLY TO YOU.** All you have to do is open your inbox and read.

☐ **EXCLUSIVE CONTENT.** We cover the news overlooked by the mainstream press.

☐ **STAY CURRENT.** Find the latest court rulings, revivals, and cultural trends.

☐ **UPDATE OTHERS.** Easy to forward to friends and family with the click of your mouse.

CHOOSE THE E-NEWSLETTER THAT INTERESTS YOU MOST:

- Christian news
- Daily devotionals
- Spiritual empowerment
- And much, much more

SIGN UP AT: **http://freenewsletters.charismamag.com**

8178